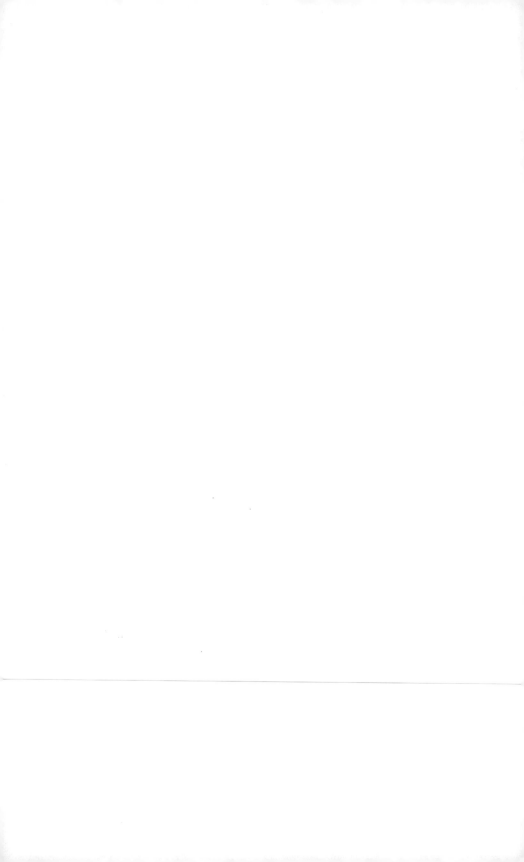

Respiratory Management of ALS
Amyotrophic Lateral Sclerosis

Lee Guion, MA, RRT, RCP
Respiratory Care Practitioner
Forbes Norris MDA/ALS Research Center
California Pacific Medical Center
San Francisco, California

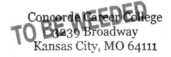

JONES AND BARTLETT PUBLISHERS
Sudbury, Massachusetts
BOSTON   TORONTO   LONDON   SINGAPORE

World Headquarters

Jones and Bartlett Publishers
40 Tall Pine Drive
Sudbury, MA 01776
978-443-5000
info@jbpub.com
www.jbpub.com

Jones and Bartlett Publishers
Canada
6339 Ormindale Way
Mississauga, Ontario L5V 1J2
Canada

Jones and Bartlett Publishers
International
Barb House, Barb Mews
London W6 7PA
United Kingdom

Jones and Bartlett's books and products are available through most bookstores and online booksellers. To contact Jones and Bartlett Publishers directly, call 800-832-0034, fax 978-443-8000, or visit our website, www.jbpub.com.

Substantial discounts on bulk quantities of Jones and Bartlett's publications are available to corporations, professional associations, and other qualified organizations. For details and specific discount information, contact the special sales department at Jones and Bartlett via the above contact information or send an email to specialsales@jbpub.com.

The authors, editor, and publisher have made every effort to provide accurate information. However, they are not responsible for errors, omissions, or for any outcomes related to the use of the contents of this book and take no responsibility for the use of the products and procedures described. Treatments and side effects described in this book may not be applicable to all people; likewise, some people may require a dose or experience a side effect that is not described herein. Drugs and medical devices are discussed that may have limited availability controlled by the Food and Drug Administration (FDA) for use only in a research study or clinical trial. Research, clinical practice, and government regulations often change the accepted standard in this field. When consideration is being given to use of any drug in the clinical setting, the healthcare provider or reader is responsible for determining FDA status of the drug, reading the package insert, and reviewing prescribing information for the most up-to-date recommendations on dose, precautions, and contraindications, and determining the appropriate usage for the product. This is especially important in the case of drugs that are new or seldom used.

Case studies are patient composites and not based on any particular patient. Names are fictitious.

Production Credits

Publisher: David Cella
Associate Editor: Maro Asadoorian
Production Director: Amy Rose
Production Supervisor: Renée Sekerak
Senior Production Editor: Susan Schultz
Production Assistant: Jill Morton

Associate Marketing Manager: Lisa Gordon
Manufacturing and Inventory Control
 Supervisor: Amy Bacus
Composition: SNP Best Set
Cover Design: Scott Moden
Printing and Binding: Malloy, Inc.
Cover printing: Malloy, Inc.

Library of Congress Cataloging-in-Publication Data
Guion, Lida.
 Respiratory management of ALS : amyotrophic lateral sclerosis / by Lida Guion.
  p. ; cm.
 Includes bibliographical references and index.
 ISBN-13: 978-0-7637-5545-4
 ISBN-10: 0-7637-5545-1
 1. Lungs—Diseases. 2. Amyotrophic lateral sclerosis. I. Title.
 [DNLM: 1. Amyotrophic Lateral Sclerosis—therapy. 2. Amyotrophic Lateral Sclerosis—complications. 3. Respiratory Insufficiency—diagnosis. 4. Respiratory Insufficiency—etiology. 5. Respiratory Insufficiency—therapy. WE 550 G964r 2009]
 RC756.G85 2009
 616.8'390636–dc22

                                                                                    2008037057
6048

Printed in the United States of America
13 12 11 10 09   10 9 8 7 6 5 4 3 2 1

Contents

Preface

There is only passing mention of ALS in most textbooks devoted to pulmonary medicine and comprehensive respiratory care. However there has been a resurgence of interest in the disease over the past 15 years due in large part to:

- Respiratory intervention, including noninvasive positive pressure ventilation (NPPV) and cough augmentation that have increased survival and reduced morbidity in people diagnosed with ALS
- Improved nutritional support, including dietary supplementation and percutaneous endoscopic gastrostomy (PEG)
- Increased understanding of the glutamine neurotransmitter system and resurgence of research
- Identification of genetic mutations in familial ALS
- Mapping of the human genome and the identification of novel genes that will inform future research in the sporadic form of the disease
- Publication of evidence-based practice parameters for managing patients with ALS
- Creation of specialized, multidisciplinary clinics in Europe and North America to provide comprehensive care for patients with ALS

The years 2005 to 2007 saw an increase in the number and scope of articles on respiratory management in ALS, notably in *Respiratory Care*, the monthly science journal of the American Association for Respiratory Care (AARC); *Chest*, journal of the American College of Chest Physicians; and *Amyotrophic Lateral Sclerosis*, the official publication of the World Federation of Neurology Research Group on Motor Neuron Diseases. A meta-analysis of the diagnosis and management of respiratory insufficiency in ALS was undertaken (Heffernan et al., 2006). An evidence-based review of current treatment practices in ALS was published in Europe (Andersen et al., 2005). The American Academy of Neurology published an update to the practice parameter for the care of patients with amyotrophic lateral sclerosis in 2008 (Miller et al., 1999). Rigorous studies have been undertaken in the respiratory management of ALS, including a randomized controlled trial of noninvasive positive pressure ventilation (Bourke et al., 2006). However, to our knowledge there is no book devoted solely to the assessment and management of respiratory symptoms in neuromuscular diseases in general, and ALS in particular.

In the multidisciplinary clinic, outpatient setting, or hospital, respiratory care practitioners (RCP) can play a pivotal role. Specialized knowledge and training in respiratory assessment, pulmonary function testing, secretion management, sleep architecture, airway care, mechanical ventilation, and noninvasive positive pressure ventilation equip RCPs to improve the quality of life and extend survival in people with ALS.

Respiratory Management of ALS provides an overview of ALS for those new to the disease and a detailed approach to the assessment of the upper and lower airway and how motor neuron loss impairs respiratory function. Treatment options emphasize symptom management and enhanced quality of life. Palliative care, decisions at end-of-life, and long-term mechanical ventilation in patients with ALS are included. Respiratory therapy students, respiratory care practitioners, nurses in neurology clinics, primary care physicians, and pulmonologists whose practice includes patients with motor neuron disease will all benefit from the review of bulbar and thoracic muscles, loss of function, and treatment recommendations.

There remains a great deal of variability in ALS evaluation and treatment (Lechtzin, 2006). Guidelines and recommendations for assessment and symptom management in *Respiratory Management of ALS* are based, whenever possible, on prospective, randomized controlled studies. When these are not available, recommendations are based on expert opinion, retrospective studies, and observational research.

Questions for future research are included at the end of each chapter in the hope readers will ask their own questions and mount studies to answer them. Respiratory care practitioners and students are encouraged to share experiences in print and at conferences. In this way we will contribute to the development of consistent and effective management of respiratory symptoms and continue to raise the standard of care in ALS.

REFERENCES

Andersen PM, Borasio GD, Dengler R, et al. EFNS task force on management of amyotrophic lateral sclerosis: guidelines for diagnosing and clinical care of patients and relatives. *Eur J Neurol* 2005;12:921–938.

Bourke, SC, Bullock RE, Williams TL, et al. Randomized controlled trial of non-invasive ventilation in amyotrophic lateral sclerosis. *ALS and Other Motor Neuron Disord* 2003;5:59.

Heffernan C, Jenkinson C, Holmes T, et al. Management of respiration in MND/ALS patients: an evidence based review. *Amyotrophic Lateral Sclerosis* 2006;7: 5–15.

Lechtzin N. Respiratory effects of amyotrophic lateral sclerosis: problems and solutions. *Resp Care* 2006;51(8):871–881.

Miller RG, Rosenberg JA, Gelinas DF, et al. Practice parameter: the care of the patient with amyotrophic lateral sclerosis (an evidence-based review): report of the Quality Standards Subcommittee of the American Academy of Neurology: ALS Practice Parameters Task Force. *Neurology* 1999;52:1311–1323.

Acknowledgments

I met my first patient with ALS when I was working in home care. She was a woman roughly my age and also in the healthcare professions. My second patient with ALS was also a woman of my generation, raising an adolescent son and recently caring for a mother with Alzheimer's disease. "But wait," I thought, "isn't ALS a disease that strikes older men?" Now that I have been working with people with ALS—PALS as many like to be known—I know that although more men are affected than women, it can strike any adult, and occasionally an adolescent. Since the cause of the sporadic form of the disease is still under investigation, any of us, including myself, may be faced with a life of progressive muscle weakness and paralysis, or we may come into contact with someone who is living with ALS, as a friend, co-worker, or as a healthcare provider.

When I began working in a multidisciplinary ALS clinic I was surprised to find no comprehensive textbook on the respiratory management of ALS. Certainly I had physicians, nurses and other RCPs with many years of experience in the field as resources. I read articles in medical journals whose conclusions, for the most part, were based on expert opinion and observational studies. Studies with small sample sizes and of short duration were the norm. There was information available about the various aspects of assessing and managing respiratory insufficiency, from distinguishing dyspnea from fatigue to the challenges of caring for a family member requiring continuous noninvasive or invasive ventilation, but this information had not been pulled together in one place.

Fortunately, Dave Cella, the editor of health professions publications at Jones and Bartlett Publishers, called to ask me to contribute a chapter about neuromuscular disease to a respiratory textbook. As we talked about what respiratory therapy students needed to know in order to work with the ALS patient population, it became clear that it was more information than one chapter could hold. Dave asked me to submit an outline for a book. My research from the past came together and it was not long after that Dave gave me the green light to pursue this project.

A book with sole authorship belies the fact that no one writes a book alone. I have had the good fortune to work with Maro Asadoorian, associate editor, who guided me through a publishing world with which I was thoroughly unfamiliar; Renée Sekerak, senior production editor; and Lisa Gordon, marketing and publicity.

It is not possible to thank everyone who has contributed to this endeavor, but some people must be recognized by name: foremost, my partner Roz Leiser, whose humor, support and patience kept me going and whose feedback helped me clarify my ideas; my colleagues at the Forbes Norris MDA/ALS Research Clinic who reviewed selected chapters, Susan Woolley-Levine, Amy Roman, and Bob Osborne; reviewers at the University of California-San Francisco, Jennifer Coggiola and Jane Pannell; Louis Boitano of the University of Washington Medical Center, all of whom offered extensive comments and suggestions; Ray Hernandez and Brian Daniel, faculty in the Respiratory Therapy Program at Skyline College; Chow Saiphanh, who brought her considerable computer skills to the project; Michelle Mendoza, who pulled together years of pulmonary function studies in ALS for my review; Dallas Forshew and members of the clinical research team; Cheryl Patterson; Jodi Bales; and finally neurologists Robert G. Miller, Jonathan S. Katz, and Catherine A. Madison, who have encouraged me in my research and practice.

I extend my greatest appreciation to people with ALS, their friends and family members who have been consistently open and generous in the face of an unrelenting disease. It is for them I wrote this book, in the hope they will receive the best care possible from knowledgeable respiratory care practitioners, whether in an outpatient clinic, hospital, or at home.

Lee Guion, MA, RRT, RCP
San Francisco, California
GuionL@sutterhealth.org

CHAPTER 1

Amyotrophic Lateral Sclerosis Overview: Definition, Epidemiology, History

CHAPTER OUTLINE

INTRODUCTION

Amyotrophic lateral sclerosis (ALS) is a progressive, heterogeneous, and fatal neurodegenerative disease. As the most common motor neuron disease (MND), it affects the pyramidal motor neurons in the brain (upper motor neurons) and spinal motor neurons or bulbar innervating neurons (lower motor neurons). Clinically, it manifests in muscle wasting and spasticity (Roland & Shneider, 2001). In the United States, the preferred term is ALS. It is often called Lou Gehrig's disease, named for the New York Yankee first baseman who died of its complications in 1941. In Europe and Australia, MND is preferred. One may also see the designation ALS/MND to identify ALS as one of the diseases of the motor neurons.

DEFINITION

Amyotrophy: muscle wasting or atrophy	
-a:	without
-myo:	muscle
-trophic:	nutrition (related to interruption of nerve supply)
Lateral:	location—occurring in the motor tracts of the lateral columns of the spinal cord
Sclerosis:	hardening

CLINICAL SUBTYPES OF MND

MNDs are those that are marked by destruction of motor neurons in the spinal cord, brainstem, or both (Roland & Shneider, 2001). ALS is one type of MND. Other diseases included in the MND category are spinal muscular atrophy types I, II, and III; progressive muscle atrophy; primary lateral sclerosis; and progressive bulbar palsy. The latter three of these diseases may remain distinct diagnoses or may progress to ALS.

Pathology of classic ALS distinguishes it from other MNDs. Losses of motor neurons in spinal cord, brainstem, and cortex with associated degeneration of corticospinal and corticobulbar tracts are seen in ALS. Other MNDs may show one or more of the previously mentioned losses and degeneration, but they lack the comprehensive nature of ALS (Strong & Rosenfeld, 2003).

CLASSIFICATION

ALS is classified into two forms: familial and sporadic. Familial ALS refers to its occurrence in first-degree blood relatives but occasionally can be cousin-to-cousin or aunt or uncle-to-niece or nephew. Sporadic ALS occurs at random, with no known family history. Familial and sporadic forms of ALS are clinically indistinguishable from one another (Strong et al., 1991).

The familial form of ALS shows an autosomal-dominant pattern of inheritance and affects between 5% and 13% of patients. Of this group 10% to 20% have mutations in the copper/zinc superoxide dismutase (SOD1) gene on chromosome 21 (Mitchell & Borsio, 2007). To date, 139 mutations have been found on chromosome 21 with differing modes of inheritance. Four other mutated genes have been identified: Alsin, Dynactin, SETX and VAPB, but occurrence of these mutations is very rare. Recently conducted genealogic studies confirm the suspicion that the percentage of people with the familial form of ALS may be higher than previously thought (Andersen, 2007; Ceroni et al., 1999).

A comprehensive scan of the human genome using Affymetrix high-density microarray technology conducted by TGen (Translational Genomics Research Institute, Phoenix, AZ) has identified more than 50 genetic abnormalities in people with sporadic ALS, 25 of which may play a significant role (Gautam & Regalado, 2006). This has given rise to new theories about causes of ALS, but its usefulness in clinical practice is many years in the future.

DIAGNOSTIC CRITERIA

The El Escorial diagnostic criteria for defining ALS was developed in the late 1980s and was revised in 1998 by the World Federation of Neurology Research Group on neuromuscular diseases subcommittee. Diagnosis remains largely clinical, and the El Escorial criteria provide some degree of objectivity. Five levels of diagnosis, based on motor neuron signs and the number of regions affected are as follows: definite, probable, probable with laboratory support (electromyography [EMG]), possible, and suspected. Disease progression and absence of sensory signs not explained by co-existing disease factors are significant in making the diagnosis of ALS (Brooks 1994; World Federation of Neurology Research Group on Motor Neuron Diseases, 1998). The region of disease onset varies among individuals. Clinical subtypes within ALS are defined by initial symptom: flail (hanging) arm, flail (hanging) leg, respiratory (lower airway), or bulbar (upper airway).

CLINICAL RATING SCALES

Several functional rating scales have been developed and used to measure ALS at baseline and to quantify progression. The ALS functional rating scale (ALSFRS) is a well-established measure of functional impairment in patients with ALS. It has been shown to be a strong predictor of survival. It is usually administered during face-to-face interviews with patients but can be administered over the phone. The ALSFRS is the most widely used rating scale in clinical trials. Scores can be generated from chart review for retrospective studies and appear to provide a reasonable estimate of scores obtained from face-to-face interviews (Lechtzin et al., 2007). The scale was revised to include respiratory questions, and this version is referred to as the ALSFRS-R.

EPIDEMIOLOGY

ALS is a complex, heterogeneous neurodegenerative disease. Its cause remains elusive, and there is currently no cure. Through epidemiology, the study of nonrandom patterns of disease occurrence, researchers hope to identify risk factors in the sporadic form of ALS.

Prevalence and Incidence

Once thought to be uncommon, ALS strikes 5,000 people in the U.S. each year. It now affects 30,000 people in the United States and another 30,000 in Europe. Geographically, sporadic ALS is fairly consistent, affecting 0.86 to 2.5 per 100,000 per year (Armon, 2003). Men are affected more often than women (1.7 per 100,000 to 1 per 100,000), but gender differences disappear after about the age of 60 years. Armon (2003) calculates that with an average life expectancy of 3 years after the symptom onset, the prevalence rate (the number of those living with the disease at a given time) can be estimated at three times the incidence rate, or approximately 6 per 100,000 at any given time.

Disease Triggers

ALS was first described in the medical literature by French neurologist and professor of anatomical pathology Jean-Martin Charcot (1825–1893). Almost 140 years later, the pathogenesis of ALS is still unknown but is now suspected of being a combination of genetic predisposition and exposure to exogenous or endogenous triggers (Roland, 2003).

Studies of endogenous triggers of motor neuron death are focused predominantly on oxidative stress and excitotoxicity. Excitotoxicity occurs when larger than normal concentrations of glutamate, an amino acid neuromodulator, cause toxicity in the central nervous system. Excitotoxins are thought to precipitate neuronal death by triggering excessive calcium influx into the motor neuron, stimulating a cascade mechanism, including free radical intermediates (Mitchell & Borsio, 2007).

Other areas of neurochemical research are protein aggregation, upregulation of microglial activity, mitochondrial dysfunction, macrophage activation, axonal transport defects, and novel proteins. Continued focus on cell biology and pathology is necessary for the development of drugs to treat ALS.

Exogenous causes remain speculative. Possible triggers under investigation are environmental toxins (lead, mercury, aluminum, herbicides, pesticides, and organophosphates) and multiple head traumas. Lifestyle factors being explored are at opposite ends of the health spectrum: tobacco smoking and regular, intense daily activity, including athletics and physically labor intensive jobs (Gonzales et al., 2007).

Age

Increasing age is a known independent risk factor for ALS. Mean and median ages at onset are 65 years. In clinical trials, the mean age at onset is 55 years. This discrepancy could be explained by referral bias and decreased survival at older ages. Incidence and mortality are linked to increased age. The highest incidence is in those 60 to 69 years old (Armon, 2003). As the population ages, we can expect the total number of people diagnosed with ALS to increase. The mean age of symptom onset is significantly lower in men than in women (Roland, 2003).

Survival

In general, of those with upper and lower motor neuron involvement, 10% to 20% survive for 5 years, and 50% survive for 3 years (Winhammer et al., 2005). Ten percent of people diagnosed with ALS may survive more than 10 years, and 5% may live approximately 20 years after diagnosis (ALS Therapy Development Institute, 2008). Reduced survival is associated with bulbar onset of ALS, a short time period between symptom onset and diagnosis, increased age, respiratory involvement, and weight loss (Stambler et al., 1998). Variants of the disease, such as flail or "hanging arms," seen almost exclusively in men, are correlated with longer life expectancy (Tysnes et al., 1994).

Interestingly, physicist Stephen Hawking has been diagnosed with ALS for more than 40 years but is the only known person to have achieved this longevity. Having lost the use of all muscles except for two fingers, he is confined to a wheelchair and uses a computer-generated speech synthesizer to communicate. He continues to teach, lecture, and publish.

The variability in longevity may be another indication that ALS is not one disease but many. Exploration of distinct genetic markers is likely to hold the key to this mystery.

Disease Clusters

Disease clusters are rare. One exception is Guam, where the environment appears to have played a significant role in the development of Western Pacific ALS. In the island's Chammaro population, dietary exposure is thought to have been the precipitating factor (Garruto, 1991). The possibility of an increased risk of ALS in Italian soccer players, marathoners, and U.S. Gulf War veterans is being explored. To date, no epidemiologic smoking gun has been identified.

Epidemiologic Research

The ALS Consortium of Epidemiological Studies encourages interdisciplinary collaboration among epidemiologists, neurologists, geneticists, toxicologists, and other scientists as they strive to identify environmental, lifestyle, and genetic factors associated with ALS (www.aces.stanford. edu). As part of this consortium, epidemiologists at Stanford University have developed an environmental risk survey to investigate possible environmental and lifestyle risks for ALS. The 50-page standardized questionnaire is administered in person or during a phone interview. The survey is being conducted through multiple educational and medical centers in the United States.

The Geneva Study (Genes and Environmental Exposure in Veterans with ALS) seeks to evaluate the combination of genetic susceptibility and environmental exposures in the risk of sporadic ALS. The Department of Veterans Affairs has established a national registry of veterans with ALS. Researchers at Duke University and the North Carolina Veterans Administration are exploring the potential of increased risk of ALS for veterans deployed to the 1990–1991 Persian Gulf War (Schmidt et al., 2008).

A national DNA registry has been proposed so that genetic materials obtained from people with ALS and controls can be stored for future research. Nonprofit organizations that support ALS research, people with ALS, their families and supporters successfully petitioned the federal government to include ALS as a reportable disease to the Centers for Disease Control and Reporting.

PUBLIC FIGURES WITH ALS

In the United States the most famous person diagnosed with ALS is Lou Gehrig, baseball's legendary New York Yankee first baseman. Gehrig was diagnosed in 1939 and died 2 years later, calling himself the "luckiest man" for the opportunities and successes he enjoyed before his illness. ALS does not observe international boundaries. Other famous persons diagnosed with the disease are Dmitri Shostakovich, Russian composer; David Niven, British actor; and Mao Tse-tung, Chinese leader (Aebischer & Kato, 2007). Charles Mingus, jazz musician and composer; Jacob Javits, United States Senator; and Dennis Day, Irish tenor, are a few more.

Augie Nieto, founder of Life Fitness and the popular stationary bike the Lifecycle, was diagnosed with ALS in his mid-40s. Frustrated by the lack of effective treatment, Mr. Nieto started the foundation Augie's Quest to raise private money for research on ALS cause and cure.

Scott Lew, a young Hollywood writer, producer, and actor, directed his first movie, *Bickford Schmeckler's Cool Ideas* (2006) from his wheelchair. *Living with Lew* (2007), directed by Adam Bardach, documents the humor and optimism Lew brings to fighting ALS and making movies. During the 2007 screenwriters' strike, he "walked" the picket line in his wheelchair using mouthpiece ventilation to assist his breathing and slogan chanting.

CLINICAL PRESENTATION

As neuron cells begin to atrophy and die, the body's muscles become weakened and fatigued. Clinical symptoms include muscle spasms or twitches, known as fasciculations, in the torso or extremities. Early loss of innervation in muscles of the extremities may manifest in tripping, stumbling, or the inability to grasp or hold onto household objects such as eating utensils, pencils, pens, and toothbrushes. If bulbar muscles, those of speech and swallowing, are involved, one may note changes in voice quality, slurred or thick speech, difficulty managing saliva (drooling), or difficulty chewing food. Initial symptoms vary among people diagnosed with ALS, but all will eventually progress to the pulmonary muscles, most notably the diaphragm, requiring ventilatory assistance. In rare instances, a patient will present with respiratory insufficiency as the primary symptom. An inability to wean a patient from mechanical ventilation in the intensive care unit should prompt consideration of ALS if other more obvious reasons have been excluded. EMG will assist in diagnosis.

People diagnosed with ALS retain sensory function—smell, touch, taste, sight and hearing. Ocular muscles and sphincter muscles of the bladder and rectum usually maintain their ability to function. Sexual function and desire are also maintained.

Until recently, clinicians and researchers thought that people with ALS retained mental clarity as well, but observed changes in personality, reason, and memory led neurologists and neuropsychologists to test for cognitive dysfunction. In a large group of patients with sporadic ALS, 50% had some degree of cognitive impairment, with 20% classified as moderate to severe. Fifteen percent of patients met criteria for frontotemporal dementia. Cognitive impairment was not correlated with depression, severity of disability, or duration of physical symptoms (Ringholz et al., 2005). These results are consistent with other frontotemporal dementia prevalence estimates. Deficits in working memory, attention, and concentration will negatively impact patients' ability to follow directions during testing and introduction to pulmonary treatments. Cognitive deficits may also decrease patients' ability to make informed decisions about treatment during the course of their disease.

CLINICAL DIAGNOSIS

There is no definitive diagnostic test for ALS. Diagnosis is made clinically by assessing function and assigning likelihood using the El Escorial (WFNALS, 1998) criteria and ruling out other possible neuromuscular diseases. Neurologists test for lower motor neuron and upper motor neuron signs in three regions of the body and make an initial diagnosis of ALS as definite, probable, probable with laboratory support (EMG), possible, or suspected (Brooks, 1994). Some researchers urge caution when using El Escorial classification, as the terminology may be confusing to patients and their families (Forbes et al., 2001).

EMG response is used to confirm a clinical diagnosis. Magnetic resonance imaging and laboratory data may be used to rule out other diseases. Laboratory tests are used to exclude diseases that can mimic ALS.

STAGES OF FUNCTIONAL DECLINE IN ALS

Denoting stages of functional decline in patients with ALS allows physicians, clinical specialists, patients, and their care providers to plan ahead and best use adaptive equipment and strategies to improve quality of life. The Mayo Clinic six-stage classification system to guide symptom management is described here (Chan & Sinaki, 1996).

- Stage I: No therapy is needed. Psychological support should be available. An exercise program should be designed to maintain muscle tone and develop auxiliary muscles while conserving energy and avoiding fatigue.
- Stage II: Patient remains ambulatory but foot drop or wrist drop because of weakness in the ankle dorsiflexors and wrist extensors, requires support with lightweight ankle–foot orthosis and wrist extension splints. Thumb-shell splints enable patients to maintain a stronger grip on items and improve hand movements.
- Stage III: Patient remains ambulatory but severe weakness may develop in ankles, wrists, hands, and neck. Patient is easily fatigued and has decreased ability in independent activities of daily living. Energy conservation is emphasized. Wheelchair is ordered. Decreased range of motion and periarthritis of the shoulder ("frozen shoulder") may occur. Stretching exercises, hydrotherapy, local heat, and massage may be prescribed.
- Stage IV: The patient is wheelchair dependent but can still perform many activities of daily living. There is severe weakness of lower extremities and moderate asymmetrical weakness of upper extremities. An electric wheelchair with adjustable height and seating and power keys for easy movement manipulation is ordered. Passive exercises are prescribed and taught to care providers. Bathroom and other home modifications are recommended.
- Stage V: Patient is dependent and wheelchair bound. Immobility puts patient at risk for skin breakdown. Care providers are instructed in turning and positioning techniques. Lifting aids, such as Hoyer, pivot, or ceiling track system, are recommended. Hospital beds are ordered with mattresses designed to avoid decubitus ulcers. Foot–ankle splints are used for positioning paralyzed lower extremities.
- Stage VI: The patient has lost all independence and is largely bedridden. Family members need assistance from extended family or home health aides in caring for patient. Swallowing and speech may be significantly impaired necessitating percutaneous endoscopic gastrostomy (PEG) and tube feedings. Respiratory muscles are impaired, requiring assistance with ventilation and secretion management. The risk of aspiration pneumonia and respiratory failure is increased. Immobility may impair urinary and bowel functions. Lower-

extremity paralysis will predispose patient to edema and thrombo-phlebitis. A risk of pulmonary embolism is increased. Most patients die of complications of respiratory muscle weakness.

Signs of respiratory muscle weakness can develop during any of the six stages. At the Mayo Clinic, the strength of respiratory muscles is moni-tored routinely and noninvasive positive pressure ventilation (NPPV) recommended when vital capacity or inspiratory pressures indicate loss of significant respiratory muscle innervation. Cough augmentation is demonstrated and mechanical insufflator-exsufflator prescribed when clinical symptoms or peak cough flow values indicate denervation of expiratory muscles and risk of secretion retention.

CLINICAL MARKERS OF RESPIRATORY DECLINE IN ALS

Care of each patient is individualized. Site of onset, disease progression, and patient response to symptoms will vary; however, in each patient, there are clinical events that mark respiratory decline and enough consis-tency among patients to allow these milestones to be useful clinically.

Markers of respiratory decline include the following:

- Shortness of breath with activity
- Need for noninvasive respiratory assistance at night because of nocturnal hypoventilation and oxygen desaturation
- Shortness of breath at rest
- Need for intermittent noninvasive respiratory assistance during the day
- Need for manual or mechanical cough assistance because of inability to mobilize secretions
- Need for continuous NPPV
- Need for decision about tracheostomy and mechanical ventilation

For most patients changes in respiratory status are gradual with a linear decline in pulmonary function measures. There may be a brief plateau and then a sudden change if lower respiratory tract infection or silent aspiration lead to pneumonia.

Without tracheostomy and mechanical ventilation, the majority of patients with ALS (86%) will die of respiratory failure (Oliver & Borasio,

2004). The majority of patients (over 90%) die peacefully. As a result of increasing hypercapnia, they become drowsy, fall into sleep, and then into a coma (Neudert et al., 2001).

Discussions among physician, patient, and family members regarding ventilatory support at the end of life should take place early in the disease course. Patients should be given all of the necessary information regarding pros and cons of tracheostomy and mechanical ventilation so that they can make informed decisions. Making their wishes known to family, friends, primary care providers, and respiratory care practitioners (RCPs) allows patients to avoid unwanted emergency intubation and ventilation. Patient and family education about the early signs and symptoms of respiratory insufficiency, silent aspiration, and pneumonia will reduce unplanned and emergent respiratory events.

DRUG TREATMENT

Clinical Trials

To date, only one drug has been approved by the U.S. Food and Drug Administration to slow the progression of ALS. Riluzole, a glutamate antagonist, has a disease-modifying effect at each stage of the disease and extends tracheostomy-free survival (Riviere et al., 1998). Riluzole is included in the practice parameter issued by the American Academy of Neurology (Miller et al., 1999). The benefits of riluzole are modest. With early administration, riluzole can extend survival for 3 to 4 months. It can be cost prohibitive for patients without a prescription drug benefit. Riluzole costs over $600 per month.

Drugs already approved by the Food and Drug Administration (FDA) to treat other diseases enable clinical trials to be conducted more quickly with ALS patients to test whether they have positive disease-modifying effects. A number of drugs have been studied in this patient population but did not have a beneficial effect on survival, disease progression, or symptoms. Ongoing and recently completed large, randomized controlled clinical trials in ALS have examined the following:

- Antibiotic *ceftriaxone*
- Antimicrobial *minocycline*
- Free radical scavenger and mitochondrial co-factor *coenzyme Q10*
- Antioxidant *selegiline*

- Antioxidant *Vitamin E (a-tocopherol)*
- Antioxidant *edaravone*
- Antioxidant *N-acetylcysteine*
- Antiexcitotoxic agent *topiramate* (antiseizure medication)
- Antiexcitotoxic agent *gabapentin* (antiglutamate strategy)
- Phosphodiesterase inhibitor *pentoxifylline*
- Mitochondrial enhancing *creatine*
- Cyclooxygenase 2 inhibitor *celecoxib*
- Ciliary neurotrophic factor *neurotrophin* (nerve growth factor)
- Neurotrophic factor *insulin-like nerve growth factor-1*

Transgenic Mouse Model

Transgenic animal models allow researchers to select drugs with potential for human trials. Over 70 drugs have been evaluated using transgenic mouse models of autosomal dominant SOD1 familial ALS. Although many drugs, including the ones listed previously here, showed promise in extending lifespan in mice, they have not shown efficacy, or caused more rapid progression of disease, in humans. The discrepancy between positive animal studies and negative clinical trial results raises doubts about the predictive values of animal studies. It should be remembered that familial ALS accounts for only 5% to 10% of all ALS cases, and SOD1 accounts for only a fifth of familial ALS.

Another challenge to investigators is determining when the disease actually begins. Approximately 50% of neurons have been lost by the time first symptoms manifest. This creates a challenge when developing treatment with neuron protective agents.

Heterogeneity

The failure of traditional pharmacotherapeutic treatments in ALS continues to frustrate researchers, patients, their families, physicians, and other healthcare providers. It now appears that clinically, biologically, and genetically ALS is a heterogeneous disease and not a single disorder (Strong, 2007). Recent DNA results have identified 25 genes suspected to play a role in ALS. Genes of interest are those involved in making "adhesion" molecules that help cells stick to one another. In ALS nerves may not be anchoring well to muscle. Another possibility is the overproduction of toxins normally beneficial to the immune system. In large amounts, toxins can damage nerve cells. Other possible genes cause degeneration of part of the skeletal muscle structure found inside motor nerves (MDA, 2006). As research into the different theories of cell damage and death expands, so should the pharmacologic approaches to treatment.

Stem Cell Therapy

Adult stem cells have been transplanted into the spinal cords of people with ALS. Although safe and well tolerated by patients when conducted in a controlled and scientific environment, stem cell therapy has not shown positive effects (Mazzini et al., 2003). Stem cell injections into transgenic mice have shown mixed results, improving survival of motor neurons while not improving clinical outcomes (Hemendinger et al., 2005). These results, although disappointing in the short run, have given researchers and patients hope for future success; however, much work needs to be done before stem cell treatment can be undertaken in experimental therapeutic trials (Mitchell & Borsio, 2007).

There are reports of U.S. citizens traveling to China for stem cell treatments at great financial expense. In Chinese stem cell treatment centers, cells of unknown type have been injected into peripheral sites, the brain, and spinal cord. Results of these treatments have not been published in peer-reviewed scientific journals, and no positive outcomes in longevity and symptom abatement have been reported. On December 19, 2007, the U.S. FDA's Office of Criminal Investigations announced the prison sentence of a New Jersey woman who falsely claimed to be able to treat ALS with stem cell therapy. The defendant and co-conspirator were convicted in December 2006 of receiving thousands of dollars in payments from unsuspecting ALS patients and their families desperate for a cure. The defendants told their patients that they had received FDA approval to treat ALS (FDA, 2007).

Lithium Trials

In February 2008, Italian researchers published results of lithium carbonate used in combination with riluzole as a treatment for ALS (Fornai et al., 2008). In this small study conducted on 44 subjects over 15 months, daily doses of lithium used in conjunction with riluzole showed that ALS progression was slowed significantly. Lithium, most commonly used to treat bipolar disorder, is known to be neuroprotective. Demonstration of increased survival rates in transgenic mouse studies led to human clinical trials. Larger multicenter safety and efficacy trials are now underway in the United States.

SYMPTOM MANAGEMENT

Although research into cause and cure has been inconclusive, symptom management has improved significantly. Great strides have been made in the areas of nutrition, communication augmentation, and respiratory intervention. Respiratory management is geared toward treating hypoventilation, resting fatigued respiratory muscles, enhancing sleep quality through improvements in sleep stage distribution, and secretion management (Simonds, 2006). The use of supportive therapies has been shown to improve survival, symptoms, and quality of life (Scott et al., 2008).

MULTIDISCIPLINARY CARE

Multidisciplinary care clinics for ALS and neuromuscular diseases are "not the end but the beginning of care" (Belsh & Schiffman, 1996). Neurology departments with a multidisciplinary team of clinical specialists not only can provide an accurate diagnosis of MND but also are able to coordinate symptom management. Individualized pharmacologic, nutritional, physical, occupational, and respiratory therapy is provided in centers that often conduct neuroscience and clinical research assuring evidence-based, state-of-the-art care. Patients should be referred to the closest multidisciplinary clinic as soon as ALS is suspected (Van den Berg et al., 2005).

Forbes Norris, MD, pioneering neurologist, working with Dee Holden Norris, RN, championed the caring approach to symptom management in ALS. Doctors Donald Mulder, Hiyashi Mitsumoto, Richard Olney, and Richard Smith, among others, developed or expanded the concept of multidisciplinary care in ALS. Today, with patient and family at the center of care, treatments are recommended and implemented based on the patient's definition of quality of life and personal experience of the disease. Continuity of care among outpatient neuromuscular clinics, community-based services, respiratory home care, primary care physicians, palliative care units, and hospices allows for flexibility and consistency in service delivery. Life expectancy and quality of life are improved through participation in multidisciplinary care clinics (Van den Berg et al., 2005).

Multidisciplinary Clinic as a Model for Care

Multidisciplinary clinics offer:

- Comprehensive care
- One-stop shopping for patients
- Team review of patients and discussion of treatment recommendations
- A site for clinical research

Multidisciplinary Team Members

Key members of the multidisciplinary team are listed here with a brief description of their role. The clinical specialists and number of team members will vary from center to center and country to country, but the primary services provided are consistent.

Neurologist

Neurologists make the diagnosis of ALS and discuss the diagnosis and its implications with the patient and family. They direct the clinic, providing clinical and scientific direction. They communicate with primary care physicians and other specialists caring for the patient. Neurologists direct medical management and are providers of record. Other members of the team provide neurologists with results of their clinical assessments and treatment recommendations. Guidelines for physicians on how to break the news of an ALS diagnosis to the patient and family are included in practice parameters of the American Academy of Neurology (Miller et al., 1999).

Nurse Specialist

Nurse specialists coordinate care provided by allied heath professionals and other team members. They act as a liaison between the patient/family and the clinic and advocate for the patient within the health care system and with insurance companies. Nurse specialists review laboratory data and medication prescriptions. They are the liaison between the ALS clinic and nurse managers on the acute-care and palliative-care units as well as with nurse specialists from home care and hospice agencies. ALS nurse specialists ensure that patients have completed an advanced directive for health care. They ensure that neurologists and clinic staff are aware of patient preferences for end-of-life care. They are responsible for following up with the physician and staff recommendations for care, such as diagnostic testing or surgical procedures. They are the "point person" in the clinic with an overview of patient and family needs.

ALS nurse specialists serve as educators to patients and families. They try to determine what patients want to know and what they need to know at any given time in the disease process. Nurse specialists work closely with neurologists to help patients and family members understand the disease process and treatment options.

ALS nurse specialists are also the bowel specialists within the multidisciplinary team. They obtain a baseline and inquire about changes in bowel patterns during each clinic visit. Many things may contribute to constipation, including decreased mobility and inactivity, decreased fluid intake with bulbar weakness, dietary changes, abdominal weakness, or medication, especially narcotics. A distended gut or abdomen will contribute to dyspnea because of displacement of the diaphragm and loss of lung capacity, and thus, RCPs should confer with the nurse specialist about changes in bowel habits.

Respiratory Care Practitioner

RCPs conduct pulmonary function tests; monitor changes in vital capacity, inspiratory pressures, and cough flow rates; and report results to neurologists, nurse specialists, and other members of the team. RCPs conduct thorough respiratory assessments at each clinic visit and recommend treatment with NPPV when indicated by patient symptoms and results of pulmonary function tests. They determine initial IPAP and EPAP settings and recommend a titration schedule. Acclimation and adherence to NPPV therapy are important roles of the RCP within the clinic. Knowledge of the range of devices that can provide NPPV and interface options is essential.

RCPs counsel patient and family on prophylaxis against respiratory infections and provide education and tools for the management of respiratory insufficiency. They provide volume expansion and secretion mobilization techniques. They instruct family members in manually assisted coughing, Heimlich and self-Heimlich maneuvers, which are reinforced by the speech language pathologist (SLP).

RCPs screen patients for signs of silent aspiration and gastroesophageal reflux disease. They may take the role of assessing oral hygiene and providing education and tools for care of teeth and gums or share this role with the nurse specialist or SLP.

In patients with moderate to severe bulbar muscle dysfunction, RCPs may counsel the patient on the pros and cons of tracheostomy for airway protection. RCPs are the clinic resource specialist for decisions about mechanical ventilation, benefits and risks, and which models are best for use in the home. RCPs serve as liaison between the ALS clinic and RCP home care specialists. They are knowledgeable about Centers for Medicare and Medicaid Service guidelines for reimbursement for respiratory equipment in the home and act as patient advocate with third party payers.

Clinic-based RCPs monitor patients to insure that NPPV or mechanical ventilation settings are effective in treating hypoxemia and hypercapnia through assessment of nocturnal oximetry or end tidal CO_2 results.

Much like their ALS nurse specialist colleagues, RCPs serve as liaisons between the neuromuscular clinic and hospital-based RCPs, many of whom have worked only rarely, if at all, with ALS patients. RCPs who specialize in neuromuscular diseases can serve as educators and be a resource to departments of respiratory care. This relationship between in-patient and outpatient services reinforces the continuum of care.

Finally, RCPs in neuromuscular clinics serve as preceptors to students in respiratory care programs. ALS care is increasingly included as a specialty rotation for graduating seniors interested in MNDs and how a multidisciplinary team functions. Many multidisciplinary ALS clinics host graduate students. Respiratory therapy students will find themselves in the company of speech language pathology and physical therapy students, fellows in neurology and pulmonary medicine, and postdoctoral students in neuropsychology.

Physical Therapist

Physical therapists (PTs) evaluate upper- and lower-extremity strength and motor function. They note symptoms of muscle stiffness, spasms, and cramps. Based on their evaluation, PTs recommend stretching exercises, energy conservation, and mobility aids and fit patients for orthoses for leg and ankle, hand, and arm. They conduct a home evaluation and recommend equipment and organization strategies that will improve patient safety and increase mobility. When the patient is no longer able to move upper or lower extremities, PTs instruct care providers in passive range of motion exercises.

Occupational Therapist

Occupational therapists (OTs) assess patient ability to perform activities of daily living and provide detailed recommendations to improve independence and functioning. In conjunction with the PTs, OTs conduct home assessments and may coordinate modifications with patient and family or make referrals to adaptability specialists. OTs design work simplification strategies and recommend techniques for energy conservation and activity modification. They may work with vendors to design and modify electric wheelchairs. They discuss with patients and families the timing of hospital beds, Hoyer lifts, and other devices to assist care providers with moving and transferring patients. They may assist patients with special needs for automobile or airline travel.

Speech Language Pathologists

SLPs evaluate patients for dysphagia (difficulty swallowing) and dysarthria (difficulty speaking). Evaluation is done through observation, palpation, and endoscopic visualization of vocal cord functioning. Word generation is recorded, and the quality of speech and volume is noted. Modified videofluoroscopy can identify swallowing difficulties and risk of aspiration. SLPs ask detailed questions about temperature and consistency of food and liquids that are difficult to manage and coughing and choking triggers. Recommendations about thickening agents, head and neck positioning during swallowing, and Heimlich and self-Heimlich maneuvers are provided.

SLPs assess patients' needs for communication augmentation devices at each stage of the disease process. These can be as simple as a call bell or as complex as a computerized eye-gaze system. Spelling boards, page turners and voice amplifiers are a few of the tools at their disposal.

Registered Dietitian

Registered dietitians (RDs) assess the nutritional status of patients during each clinic visit. Dietitians often work closely with SLPs to assess swallowing impairment. Dietitians note the patient's weight at each clinic visit and recommend strategies to maintain weight and increase caloric intake. They discuss consistency of food, its protein, fat, and carbohydrate composition, and may provide recipes in conjunction with energy conservation strategies during food preparation and eating. Liquid dietary supplements are encouraged. If patients are at risk for malnutrition due to bulbar weakness, dietitians, in conjunction with the nurse and neurologist, will discuss enteral feeding. If the patient chooses to undergo PEG or radiologically inserted gastrostomy, dietitians will determine the patient's caloric needs and prescribe a formula to meet them. Dietitians will often demonstrate the initial PEG feeding postoperatively and teach care providers how to manage the feeding tube. The dietitian or nurse will monitor the PEG site on subsequent clinic visits for signs of irritation or infection.

Social Worker

Social workers often serve as counselors and family therapists, helping the patient and family to adjust to and accept the diagnosis of ALS. Their knowledge of community resources is invaluable to families overwhelmed by sudden changes in finances and relationships, the need for in-home support services, the care of children or aging parents, and future planning. Social workers assist patients applying for Medicare or Medicaid health benefits, filling our disability forms, or seeking alternative housing. Social workers may also serve as counselors to the multidisciplinary team whose members experience loss on a continual basis as new patients face disability and established clinic patients face death.

Neuropsychologist

Neuropsychologists integrate knowledge of brain function and behavior. They conduct a multidimensional examination through which they assess ALS patients for clinical and behavioral signs of cognitive impairment. They assess executive function, word retrieval, word generation, visual–spatial abilities, apathy, and empathy. Neuropsychologists can distinguish between depression, psychoses, and dementia and determine which are treatable and which are not. This information is important to all members of the team because a patient's cognition will impact their ability to follow instructions and make important decisions about care.

ALS Association and Muscular Dystrophy Association

The ALS Association (ALSA) and Muscular Dystrophy Association (MDA) offer financial support to many multidisciplinary neuromuscular clinics throughout the United States. This support helps defray the costs of home visits and expensive medical equipment for patients who lack insurance or full coverage. ALSA and MDA representatives are considered part of the multidisciplinary team and are encouraged to meet with patients and family members to inform them of the range of services their organizations provide. Money raised by ALSA and MDA directly supports patients, raises awareness of the disease, and provides funds for scientific research into cause and cure.

Other members of the multidisciplinary team may include the following:

- Designated pulmonologist
- Designated gastroenterologist
- EMG technician
- Medical assistant
- Administrative staff
  - Manager
  - Receptionist
  - Insurance verification specialist
  - Billing specialist

Role of the RCP in Clinical Research

Multidisciplinary teams bring an opportunity to participate in original research. Although standards of care in ALS are being sought through evidence-based guidelines, treatments are often based on expert opinion or observational research, and vary internationally (Andersen et al., 2005; Heffernan et al., 2006, Miller et al., 1999). A cure for ALS is many years off; therefore, a major focus of research is symptom control and quality of life. There are many areas in which RCPs can contribute to best practice in the respiratory management of ALS.

TOPICS FOR RESEARCH

- The best pulmonary function test to determine early respiratory compromise in clinically asymptomatic patients
- A comparison of pulmonary function tests to determine best diagnostic test for respiratory insufficiency in patients with moderate-to-severe bulbar symptoms

- The best methods of identifying silent aspiration
- Techniques to improve acceptance of and adherence to NPPV in patients who are asymptomatic or only mildly symptomatic
- Noninvasive ventilator modalities and options that are most beneficial for people with ALS
- Factors that predict tracheostomy and mechanical ventilation choice when patients are faced with impending respiratory failure

SUMMARY

ALS was first described in the mid-1800s. Since that time, genetic research has allowed investigators to identify a familial form of the disease and genetic markers that may predispose people to developing the sporadic form. It is now generally recognized that ALS is a heterogeneous disease, and thus, research into its etiology and treatment must be multipronged. Drugs to modify the course of ALS are being sought; however, recent advances in symptom management, especially respiratory failure and malnutrition, have increased the lifespan and quality of life of people with ALS.

Palliation, the relief of symptoms and improved quality of life, is the focus in ALS care. RCPs have an important role to play in the management of dyspnea, nocturnal hypoventilation, and reduced vital capacity. RCPs provide comfort to patients and families by explaining the options at end of life. Specialized training in respiratory assessment and treatment make the RCP an important clinical resource within the multidisciplinary team.

REFERENCES

Aebischer P, Kato A. Playing defense against Lou Gehrig's Disease. *Scientific American* November 2007;86–93.

Affymetrix Inc. Available at www.affymetrix.com.

ALS Therapy Development Institute, Cambridge, MA. World's largest research and development program focused exclusively on ALS; 2008. Available at www.als.net.

Andersen P. Genetics of ALS/MND and the role of modifier genes: a clinical perspective. *Amyotrophic Lateral Sclerosis* 2007;8(Suppl 1):7–8.

Andersen P, Borasio GD, Dengler R, et al. EFNS task force on management of amyotrophic lateral sclerosis: guidelines for diagnosing and clinical care of patients and relatives: and evidenced-based review with good practice points. *Eur J Neurol* 2005;12:921–938.

Armon C. Epidemiology of amyotrophic lateral sclerosis/motor neuron disease. In Shaw P, Strong M (eds.). *Motor Neuron Disorders.* Philadelphia: Butterworth & Heinemann; 2003, pp. 167–206.

Bardach A, Living with Lew 2007. www.imdb.com/title/tt0947044/

Belsh JM, Schiffman PL (eds.). *Amyotrophic Lateral Sclerosis: Diagnosis and Management for the Clinician.* Armonk, NY: Futura Publishing Co.; 1996, p. xi.

Brooks BR. El Escorial World Federation of Neurology Criteria for the Diagnosis of Amyotrophic Lateral Sclerosis. *J Neurol Sci* 1994;124(Suppl):96–107.

Ceroni M, Malaspina A, Poloni TE, et al. Clustering of ALS patients in central Italy due to the occurrence of the L84F SOD1 gene mutation. *Neurology* 1999; 53:1064–1071.

Chan CW, Sinaki M. Rehabilitation management of the ALS patient. In Belsh JM, Schiffman PL (eds.). *Amyotrophic Lateral Sclerosis: Diagnosis and Management for the Clinician.* Armonk, NY: Futura Publishing Co.; 1996.

FDA investigation leads to prison sentence for woman who claimed to cure "Lou Gehrig's Disease." Press release December 19, 2007. U.S. Food and Drug Administration, Department of Health and Human Services. Available at www.fds.gov/bbs/topics/NEWS/2007/NEW01760. Accessed December 28, 2007.

Forbes RB, Colville S, Swingler RJ. Are the El Escorial and revised El Escorial criteria for ALS reproducible? A study of inter-observer agreement. *Amyotrophic Lateral Sclerosis Other Motor Neuron Disord* 2001;2:135–138.

Fornai F, Longone P, Cafaro L, et al. Lithium delays progression of amyotrophic lateral sclerosis. *PNAS* 2008;105:2052–2057.

Garruto RM. Pacific paradigms of environmentally-induced neurological disorders: clinical, epidemiological and molecular perspectives. *Neurotoxicology* 1991;12:347–377.

Gautam N, Regalado A. Trail of a killer: a fitness mogul, stricken by illness hunts for genes. *Wall Street Journal* November 30, 2006:1:12.

Gonzales A, Morales R, Pageot N, et al. ALS patients have a significant hyperactivity at all ages: results of a prospective study. *Amyotrophic Lateral Sclerosis* 2007;8(Suppl 1):67–68.

Heffernan C, Jenkinson C, Holmes T, et al. Management of respiration in MND/ALS patients: an evidence based review. *Amyotrophic Lateral Sclerosis* 2006; 7:5–15.

Hemendinger R, Wang J, Malik S, et al. Sertoli cells improve survival of motor neurons in SOD1 transgenic mice, a model of amyotrophic lateral sclerosis. *Exp Neurol* 2005;196:235–243.

Lechtzin N, Kimball R, Busse A, et al. The accuracy of ALSFRS scores calculated from retrospective review of clinical notes. *Amyotrophic Lateral Sclerosis* 2007; 8(Suppl 1):139.

Lew, S. Bickfordmovie.com 2006 http://www.indb.com/name/nm/0506712/

Mazzini L, Fagioli F, Noccaletti R, et al. Stem cell therapy in amyotrophic lateral sclerosis: a methodological approach in humans. *Amyotrophic Lateral Sclerosis Other Motor Neuron Disord* 2003;4:158–161.

MDA Press Release. Scan of entire human genome finds unexpected new clues on Lou Gehrig's disease. November 30, 2006. www.mda.org/publications/resdev. html and http://www.medicalnewstoday.com/articles/78567.php

Miller RG, Rosenberg JA, Gelinas DF, et al. Practice parameter: the care of the patient with amyotrophic lateral sclerosis (an evidence-based review): report of the Quality Standards Subcommittee of the American Academy of Neurology: ALS Practice Parameters Task Force. *Neurology* 1999;52:1311–1323.

Mitchell JD, Borsio GD. Amyotrophic lateral sclerosis. *Lancet* 2007;369:2031–2041.

Neudert C, Oliver D, Wasner M, et al. The course of the terminal phase in patients with amyotrophic lateral sclerosis. *J Neurol* 2001;248:612–616.

Oliver D, Borasio GD. Disease of the motor nerves. In Voltz R, Vernat JL, Borasio GD, el al. (eds.). *Palliative Care in Neurology*. Oxford, UK: Oxford University Press; 2004.

Ringholz GM, Appel SH, Bradshaw M, Cooke NA, Mosnik DM, Schulz PE. Prevalence and patterns of cognitive impairment in sporadic ALS. *Neurology* 2005;65:586–590.

Riviere M, Meininger V, Zeisser P, Munsat T. An analysis of extended survival in patients with amyotrophic lateral sclerosis with riluzole. *Arch Neurol* 1998;55:526–528.

Roland LR. Clinical aspects of sporadic amyotrophic lateral sclerosis. In Shaw P, Strong M (eds.). *Motor Neuron Disorders*. Philadelphia: Butterworth & Heinemann; 2003, pp. 111–143.

Roland LR, Shneider N. Amyotrophic lateral sclerosis. *N Engl J Med* 2001;344:1688–1700.

Schmidt S, Allen KD, Loiacono VT, et al. Genes and environmental exposure in veterans with amyotrophic lateral sclerosis: the GENEVA study. *Neuroepidemiology* 2008;30:191–204.

Scott S, Kraus J, Cole J, et al. Design, power and interpretation of studies in the standard murine model of ALS. *Amyotrophic Lateral Sclerosis* 2008;9:4–15.

Simonds A. Recent advances in respiratory care for neuromuscular disease. *Chest* 2006;130:1879–1886.

Stambler N, Charatan M, Lederbaum JM. Prognostic indicators of survival in ALS: ALS CNTF Treatment Study Group. *Neurology* 1998;50:66–72.

Strong M. ALS: one disease or many? *Amyotrophic Lateral Sclerosis* 2007;8(Suppl 1):7–8.

Strong M, Rosenfeld J. Amyotrophic lateral sclerosis: a review of current concepts. *ALS Other Motor Neuron Disord* 2003;4:136–143.

Strong M, Hudson AJ, Alvord WG. Familial amyotrophic lateral sclerosis, 1850–1989: a statistical analysis of the world literature. *Can J Neurol Sci* 1991;18:45–58.

Translational Genomics Research Institute (TGen). Available at www.tgen.org.

Tysnes OB, Vollset SE, Larsen JP, Aarli JA. Prognostic factors and survival in amyotrophic lateral sclerosis. *Neuroepidemiology* 1994;13:226–235.

Van den Berg JP, Kalmijn S, Lindeman E, et al. Multidisciplinary ALS care improves quality of life in patients with ALS. *Neurology* 2005;65:1264–1267.

Winhammer JM, Rowe DB, Henderson RD, Kierman MC. Assessment of disease progression in motor neuron disease. *Lancet Neurol* 2005;4:229–238.

World Federation of Neurology Research Group on Motor Neuron Diseases. *El Escorial Revisited: Revised Criteria for the Diagnosis of Amyotrophic Lateral Sclerosis.* ALS Consensus Conference, Airlie House, Warrington, Virginia, 1998. Available at www.wfnals.org.

Neuroanatomy and Respiratory Physiology

CHAPTER OUTLINE

INTRODUCTION

In March 2006, a multidisciplinary group of pulmonologists, neurologists, intensivists, anesthesiologists, and respiratory therapists gathered in Ixtapa, Mexico. The occasion for this gathering was the 37th *Respiratory Care* Journal Conference, the first time the American Association for Respiratory Care (2006) had brought together neurology and pulmonary specialists to discuss and debate respiratory dysfunction and treatment options in neuromuscular disease. In January 2007, the Amyotrophic Lateral Sclerosis Association (ALSA) brought together neurologists, pulmonologists, surgeons, and respiratory therapists at the Will Rogers Symposium in Newport Beach, California. The significance of these professional meetings was the coming together of neurology and pulmonary medicine to discuss respiratory insufficiency in neurologic disease and neurologic causes of chronic respiratory failure in amyotrophic lateral sclerosis (ALS).

The introductory lecture at both historic meetings was the neurorespiratory system. This is where we begin our tour of ALS.

FUNCTIONAL NEURORESPIRATORY ANATOMY

Understanding the pathway from brain to muscle is essential to knowing ALS and its clinical consequences. The flow of information from brain to muscle is initiated in the cerebral cortex, where voluntary breathing is controlled. The brainstem, spinal cord, motor neurons, and respiratory muscles work in a feedback system that controls automatic breathing.

Cortex ⇒ Brainstem ⇒ Spinal cord ⇒ Nerve root ⇒
Peripheral nerve ⇒ Neuromuscular junction ⇒ Respiratory muscle

Between the brainstem and the respiratory muscles, chemoreceptors (those responding to O_2, CO_2, and H^+) and neuroreceptors (slowly adapting, rapidly adapting, and C-fiber receptors) control breathing and respiration. In 1868, Hering and Breuer discovered the mechanics of stretch receptors and reflex control in breathing. They noted that lung inflation signaled the end of inhalation and that lung deflation triggered inhalation while suppressing exhalation (Figure 2-1). For voluntary movement, the

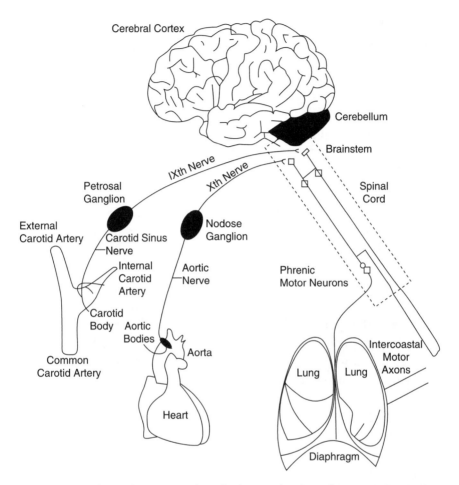

FIGURE 2-1 Chemical Receptors and Feedback Loops that Control Automatic Respiration. Physiology of Respiration, 2E (2001) by Hlastala, Michael & Berger, Albert. By permission of Oxford University Press, Inc.

motor cortex directs the muscle movement desired, whereas the cerebellum monitors the muscle movement by comparing intended movement with actual movement. The cerebellum and motor cortex communicate to fine tune movement.

The peripheral nervous system consists of cranial and spinal nerves. The central nervous system consists of brain and spinal cord. The brain, in turn, consists of cerebrum and brain stem. The brain stem components include the midbrain, pons, cerebellum, and medulla. The cerebrum contains the cortex. The cerebral cortex is the layer of grey matter covering the entire surface of the brain. ("Cortical" refers to the cerebral cortex.) In functional terms the cortex is divided into the motor cortex, sensory cortex, and association cortex. It is the motor cortex that we are concerned with here.

PATHOBIOLOGY

Cerebral Cortex

The cerebral cortex controls the majority of the neuronal "traffic" that originates in and passes through the brainstem. This includes the descending motor pathways. This pathway includes the upper motor neurons (UMNs) and lower motor neurons (LMNs). In the classic description of neuropathology in ALS, UMNs of the brain's motor cortex talk to the LMNs of the brainstem and throughout the spinal cord via the corticospinal tracts (Hirano, 1982; Strong & Rosenfeld, 2003). The LMN exits the spinal cord and becomes the spinal nerve roots and the nerves that supply respiratory muscles. When the nerves reach the muscle, they begin dividing, first into "twigs" and then into "boutons" that attach themselves like suction cups to the muscle membrane and release acetylcholine with each nerve firing into the junction between nerve and muscle (the synapse). The neurotransmitter (acetylcholine) binds to receptors (end plates) on the muscle side of the junction. This action depolarizes the muscle membrane and ultimately results in muscle fiber contraction (Benditt, 2006).

It now appears that the first signs of motor neuron degeneration occur not in the cell body, but at the synaptic junction, specifically the synaptic terminal and the axon. Long axons transport energy-generating mitochondria and growth factors between the cell body and the synaptic terminal. When this transportation system breaks down, motor neurons die (Aebischer & Kato, 2007). What neurologists see during neurologic and motor examination of a patient is severe weakness, hyperreflexia, increased tone, the presence of Babinski signs, spasticity, and clonus indicating UMN degeneration. Weakness, atrophy, flaccidity, muscle cramping, fasciculations, and, with medullary involvement, dysarthria and dysphagia are seen with LMN degeneration. These physical finding plus diffuse neurologic changes and fibrillations on EMG, lead to a positive diagnosis of ALS.

Spinal Cord

ALS is a motor neuron-selective process marked by degeneration of the descending spinal pathway serving motor function. In ALS, destruction of the anterior horn cells of the motor neurons in the spinal cord, Betz cell loss, and pyramidal tract degeneration lead to respiratory muscle weakness, atrophy, and eventual paralysis (Mier, 1990). Cell death occurs both where cells proliferate in the neuroepithelium and migrating neuroblasts and later where they differentiate at synaptic junctions (Przedborski & Clark, 2003). On autopsy, surviving motor neurons of the anterior horn cells exhibit three stages of death. Cells in these stages have been described as (1) normal in appearance except swollen and round with nucleus eccentrically placed; (2) cell body shrunken with hazy multipolar shape and blebbing, with nucleus homogeneous and condensed; and (3) motor neuron shrunken to 20% of its normal size, cell body rounded, and devoid of any process with nucleus extremely condensed (Przedborski & Clark). This final stage is called the apoptotic stage, a term that is used to describe cell deletion by a fragmentation process in which its particles are ingested by other cells (phagocytosed).

NEURODEGENERATIVE ACTION

Much of the research in ALS is focused on which molecules might signal and amplify the neurodegenerative action leading to motor neuron death. Once thought to be distinct processes, in recent years, the "metabolic turmoil" in ALS is seen to be the interrelationship among the biochemical disturbances of the motor neuron: inflammatory free radicals produced within the motor neuron, levels of oxidative metabolism, protein aggregates, glutamate-induced excitotoxicity, mitochondrial dysfunction, intermediate filament metabolism, and molecular pathways (Strong, 2007). Genetic predisposition, or accumulative damage through the aging process, may be triggered or aggravated by endogenous or exogenous agents.

In the face of this cascade of cell death, some degree of respiratory muscle involvement can be detected even before respiratory symptoms develop. Fifty percent of nerve cells may have been lost before detection of initial symptoms. Because healthy respiratory muscles harbor considerable reserves, significant weakness may occur before it is seen in abnormal pulmonary function testing (Mier, 1990).

COGNITIVE IMPAIRMENT IN ALS

Extraneuronal Degeneration and Cognitive Impairment

Neuropathology in ALS has traditionally focused on UMNs responsible for descending supraspinal innervation and the LMNs responsible for innervation of the skeletal muscles; however, neural injury in ALS is now recognized to extend beyond the motor system. Degeneration of the posterior columns and resulting cognitive impairment are present in a subgroup of patients with ALS (Lomen-Hoerth et al., 2003). In fact, cognitive impairment may represent a point along the disease continuum (Ringholz et al., 2005; Wilson et al., 2001) and may indicate an integral symptom of the disease itself (Strong & Rosenfeld, 2003). Cognitive impairment has been associated with neuronal loss in the frontal cortex, anterior horn cells, frontal gyral atrophy, microvaculation of temporal regions, and gliosis of frontal subcortical white matter (Ringholz et al.).

Symptoms of Cognitive Impairment

Neurologists and neuropsychologists may administer tests of fluency, oral word association, memory, and visuospatial functioning. Symptoms of cognitive impairment include a loss of decision-making skills, insight, verbal fluency, attention, and working memory. Typically, patients with ALS do not have problems with memory, but if they cannot attend well, they may appear to have memory deficits. In actuality, they simply cannot track conversations or information well. Symptoms of behavioral impairment include alterations in social comportment (apathy, agitation, loss of empathy) and personal conduct (disinhibition, impulsivity, violations of personal space) (Grossman et al., 2007).

The site of pathology affects clinical manifestations of cognitive impairment. The left brain gives us context, ego, time, and logic (Kaufman, 2008). Left frontal lobe abnormality produces apathy, aphasia, poor word generation, and reduced ability to perform dual tasks (Grossman et al., 2007). The right brain gives us creativity and empathy (Kaufman). Right frontal lobe abnormalities produce disinhibition, loss of insight, perseveration, irritability, and euphoria (Grossman et al.).

Frontotemporal Dementia

More severe impairment consistent with frontotemporal dementia (FTD) may be seen in as many 30% (Strong et al., 1999) to 50% (Lomen-Hoerth et al., 2003) of patients diagnosed with ALS; however, controlled studies suggest a much lower prevalence of dementia in ALS patients. Early anatomical lesions of FTD are seen in orbitofrontal, superior medial frontal, and anterior temporal lobes. Specific neuropsychological testing and cognitive screening techniques can identify FTD and distinguish it from other cognitive disorders, such as depression, dementia, or pseudobulbar affect, which is also referred to as inappropriate emotional expressive disorder. Clinical presentation of FTD varies, and behavioral abnormalities are not well defined. The Frontal Systems Behavioral Scale has been used to assess behavioral changes caused by apathy, disinhibition, and executive function (Grossman et al., 2007). Caregivers may complete other questionnaires describing patient behavior, such as the Neuropsychiatric Inventory (Cummings et al., 1994) and Frontal Behavioral Inventory (Kertesz et al., 1997).

Clinical Implications of Cognitive Impairment

Results of cognitive and behavioral assessments are useful to clinicians who work with ALS. If changes in cognition are suspected, respiratory care practitioners (RCPs) need to ask themselves these questions and discuss implications with other members of the multidisciplinary team:

- Is the patient able to provide an accurate medical history and description of respiratory symptoms?
- Is the patient able to grasp the respiratory implications of declining vital capacity and other measures of lung function?
- Is the patient able to understand and recall instructions for respiratory assistive devices?
- Is the patient able to follow instructions for pulmonary function testing?
- Is the patient able to make informed decisions regarding acceptance of palliative treatments such as noninvasive positive pressure ventilation, percutaneous endoscopic gastrostomy, or mechanical ventilation?
- Is the patient able to participate fully in discussions regarding end-of-life care?

Respiratory Compromise and Cognitive Function

Respiratory insufficiency directly affects brain functioning. Two studies comparing forced vital capacity (FVC) and cognitive function in ALS found a positive correlation (Woolley & Katz, 2008). In ALS patients grouped by FVC, those with lower FVCs had significantly lower scores in memory retention, retrieval efficiency, and verbal fluency. In a second study, patients diagnosed with ALS-FTD had significantly lower mean FVC (66%) compared with ALS patients without FTD (mean FVC, 99%). Noninvasive positive pressure ventilation has been shown to significantly improve cognitive function over 6 weeks in patients with ALS with reduced respiratory muscle strength and nocturnal hypoventilation (Newsom-Davis et al., 2001).

Chronic hypoventilation, hypercapnia and hypoxia may result in cognitive impairment. Altered frontal and parietal cerebral perfusion has been seen in patients with chronic obstructive pulmonary disease (COPD) with cognitive impairment (Woolley & Katz, 2008). Chronic respiratory insufficiency in motor neuron disease bears further study as frontal-type cognitive decline with hypoxemia in COPD looks similar to that found in ALS.

NEUROCHEMISTRY OF THE PULMONARY SYSTEM

Central and Peripheral Chemoreceptors

The control of breathing is both chemical and mechanical. Although the mechanisms are not completely understood, we know that central and peripheral chemoreceptors control breathing (Figure 2-2). Central chemoreceptors respond to carbon dioxide and cerebrospinal fluid pH. Peripheral receptors of the aortic and carotid bodies sense the levels of PaO_2 and to a lesser extent $PaCO_2$ and pH. A fall in PaO_2 to below 75 mm Hg (hypoxic threshold) (Burton & Kazemi, 2000) or below 60 mm Hg (Siobal, 2007) stimulates ventilation via impulses carried from the carotid bodies through the IX cranial nerve to the nucleus tractus solitarius where neurotransmitters are released. Hypercapnia accentuates ventilatory response to hypoxia with concomitant tachycardia. Ventilation, perfusion, and respiration allow oxygen to be carried from the upper airway to the level of the cells, fueling energy, and appeasing the carotid bodies. Carbon dioxide, the waste

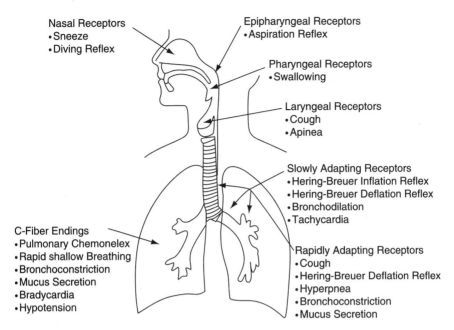

FIGURE 2-2 Mechanical Receptors Involved in Respiratory Feedback. Physiology of Respiration, 2E (2001) by Hlastala, Michael & Berger, Albert. By permission of Oxford University Press, Inc.

product of energy metabolism, is removed and exhaled. The Haldane effect shifts the O_2 dissociation curve to the left, increasing the affinity of Hb for CO_2 as O_2 is released at the tissue sites. This shift is reversed in the pulmonary capillaries so that CO_2 can be excreted from the lungs. Stretch receptors in the lung and chest wall signal end of inspiration at high lung volumes and, through communication with inspiratory centers in the medulla, allow for cycle to exhalation (Hlastals & Berger, 1996).

Neural Receptors

Neural receptors are present in the upper and lower airways, respiratory muscles, lungs, and pulmonary vessels. They include the nasal receptors (sneeze), epipharyngeal receptors (aspiration reflex), pharyngeal receptors (swallowing), and laryngeal receptors (cough). They also include the slowly adapting stretch receptors (Hering-Breuer reflex, bronchodilation), rapidly adapting receptors (bronchoconstriction, cough, mucus secretion), and C-fiber endings (pulmonary chemoreflexes, bronchoconstriction, mucus secretion) (Figure 2-1). Their activation signals the central respiratory centers via the vagus nerve (Benditt, 2006). They respond to changes in lung volume, exogenous irritants (pollen, dust, animal dander), and endogenous chemical stimuli (histamines, prostaglandins).

Pneumotaxic and Medullary Centers

The pneumotaxic center (located in the pons and also known as the pontine respiratory group [PRG]) and medullary center control the breathing pattern and respiratory rhythm. The rhythmic firing of neurons in the medulla acts as a respiratory "pacemaker" for the respiratory system by sending messages to the anterior horn cells of the motor neurons that supply the respiratory muscles. The nerve-fiber tracts that control voluntary and automatic breathing run separately within the spinal cord, where they transmit impulses to the LMNs (Figure 2-3). The LMNs exit the spinal cord and become the spinal nerve roots and nerves that supply the respiratory muscles. The chemical transmitter acetylcholine is released with nerve firing, leading to muscle fiber contraction (Benditt, 2006). The two groups of neurons that control breathing, the dorsal respiratory group (DRG) and ventral respiratory group (VRG), receive input from respiratory centers in the medulla. The dorsal respiratory group processes initial information coming from peripheral sensors through cranial nerves IX and X, whereas the ventral respiratory group projects to the motor neurons controlling accessory, abdominal, and intercostals muscles. The apneustic center in the lower pons and pneumotaxic center in the upper pons appear to play a role in moving from inspiration to exhalation (Berger et al., 1977).

INNERVATION OF RESPIRATORY MUSCLES

Different muscle groups contribute directly or indirectly to ventilation in the patient with motor neuron disease and are grouped into three areas:

- Muscles of inspiration
- Muscles of exhalation
- Muscles of the upper airway

Muscles of Inspiration

Diaphragm and Intercostals

The diaphragm is the major muscle of inspiration, providing between 70% and 80% of vital capacity in normal individuals. The diaphragm is

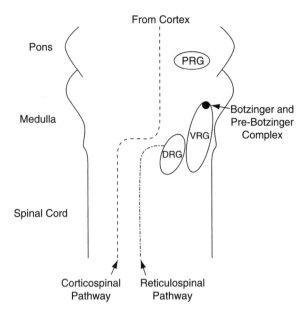

FIGURE 2-3 Brainstem and Upper Spinal Cord. Reprinted with Permission from *Respiratory Care* and the American Association for Respiratory Care: Benditt JO. The Neuromuscular Respiratory System: Physiology, Pathophysiology, and a Respiratory Care Approach to Patients. *Respir Care* 2006;51(8):829–837.

innervated by the phrenic nerve, located at level 3 through level 5 of the cervical spine. Intercostal muscles contribute to inspiration and exhalation. They are located in the intercostal spaces between the ribs and are innervated by the intercostal nerves located at the level of the thoracic spine T1–T12. There are two sheets of muscle fibers. The external intercostals contribute to inspiration by expanding the rib cage. Internal intercostals contribute to exhalation through contraction. The abdominal muscles T7–T12, L1 contribute to exhalation and stabilization of the thorax.

Accessory Muscles

Accessory muscles come into play as needed during exercise or respiratory distress or when the diaphragm and intercostal muscles are weakened by disease and no longer able to handle the work of ventilation. These include sternocleidomastoid C2–C3, scalene C4–8, trapezii C3–C4, and pectoralis major and minor, latissimus dorsi, and platysma. These muscles assist in chest expansion by moving the rib cage upward when a poorly innervated diaphragm cannot drop downward and ribcage expand outward. Chronic use of accessory muscles for ventilation results in reduced tidal volumes, increased work of breathing, fatigue, and increased metabolic energy expenditure. This in turn contributes to dyspnea, fatigue, and unintended weight loss.

In the absence of pulmonary or neuromuscular disease, breathing accounts for only 1% to 2% of total oxygen consumption. This percentage rises to 15 in diseases that require a high level of ventilation (spinal and chest wall deformities, COPD, fibrosis, and acute pneumonia). In patients with ALS who have reduced overall energy expenditure because of a loss of mobility, oxygen consumption is decreased, whereas energy expenditure for breathing can exceed 15% of total consumption (Bach, 2002).

A loss of elastic recoil when the diaphragm and intercostal muscles are impaired may result in increased residual exhaled volume and hypercapnia. Compensated hypercarbic respiratory failure occurs in a subset of people with ALS. Although this has not been explored in detail in the medical literature, students and clinicians must be aware of the possibility of carbon dioxide retention and the risk to this population if receiving supplemental oxygen without invasive or noninvasive ventilatory support.

Muscles of Exhalation

Abdominal Muscles

Abdominal muscles (internal and external obliques, rectus abdominus, and transverse abdominus) play a role during exhalation by moving the abdominal wall inward and the diaphragm upward into the thoracic cage. The rectus abdominus together with the obliques also assist exhalation by moving the lower rib cage downward and increasing pleural pressure. Compensatory paradoxical movement of the abdominal muscles (inward on inhalation) is a sign of diaphragmatic weakness and respiratory insufficiency. One may use contraction of the abdominal muscles to push the diaphragm upward forcefully, storing elastic recoil in the chest wall and assisting the subsequent inspirations (Benditt, 2006). Abdominal displacement ventilation (Pneumobelt, Respironics, Murraysville, PA) has been used with limited success by patients with diaphragmatic muscle weakness caused by muscular dystrophies.

Muscles of the Upper Airway

Upper airway muscles of the tongue, soft palate, and abductors of the vocal cords are necessary for airway patency. A loss of innervation by the cranial nerves that feed them (V, VII, IX, X, XI, and XII) (Benditt, 2006) may lead to upper airway obstruction and the need for intervention to allow for spontaneous breathing. A loss of upper airway protection because of loss of innervation of the glossopharyngeus (IX), vagus (X), glossopharyngeus (XII), and accessory (XI) nerves also puts one at risk for aspiration of saliva, liquids, and food particles. People with ALS are at risk for aspiration pneumonia, as cough and secretion removal will also be impaired by abdominal and respiratory muscle weakness.

SUMMARY

Neuromuscular respiratory failure results from a combination of factors: inspiratory muscle weakness and impaired ventilation, expiratory muscle weakness and reduced ability to cough, and upper airway muscle weakness and the risk of aspiration. Detailed knowledge of where muscle denervation occurs and its implications can guide intervention and inform a dialogue among patient, clinician, and family members about treatment options. Respiratory assessment and pulmonary function testing for the presence of neuromuscular and pulmonary compromise are the role of RCPs as is the proactive approach to prevention of acute pulmonary complications and treatment of chronic respiratory insufficiency. Subsequent chapters explore in detail respiratory assessment and management of those with ALS based on current knowledge of neurological impairment of breathing and treatment options.

REFERENCES

Aebischer P, Kato C. Playing defense against Lou Gehrig's disease. *Scientific American* November 2007:86–93. Available at www.SciAm.com.

American Association for Respiratory Care. *Respiratory Care* Journal Conference: neuromuscular disease in respiratory and critical care medicine. *Respiratory Care* 2006;51:8–9.

Bach J. Physiology and pathophysiology of hypoventilation: ventilatory vs. oxygenation impairment. In Bach J (ed.). *Noninvasive Mechanical Ventilation.* Philadelphia: Hanley & Belfus; 2002, pp. 29–30.

Benditt JO. The neuromuscular respiratory system: physiology, pathophysiology, and a respiratory care approach to patients. *Respir Care* 2006;51:829–837.

Berger AJ, Mitchell RA, Severinghaus JW. Regulation of respiration. *N Engl J Med* 1977;297:92–97, 138–143, 194–201.

Burton MD, Kazemi H. Neurotransmitters in central respiratory control. *Respir Physiol* 2000;122:111–121.

Cummings JL, Mega M, Gray K, et al. The neuropsychiatric inventory: comprehensive assessment of psychopathology in dementia. *Neurology* 1994;44: 2308.

Grossman A, Woolley-Levine S, Bradley W, Miller RG. Detecting neurobehavioral changes in amyotrophic lateral sclerosis. *Amyotrophic Lateral Sclerosis* 2007;8: 56–61.

Hirano A. Aspects of the ultrastructure of amyotrophic lateral sclerosis. *Adv Neurol* 1982;36:75–88.

Hlastals MP, Berger AJ. *Physiology of Respiration.* New York: Oxford University Press; 1996, pp. 162–208.

Kaufman L. A superhighway to bliss. *New York Times* May 25, 2008:1.

Kertesz A, Davidson W, Foz H. Frontal behavioral inventory: diagnostic criteria for frontal lobe dementia. *Can J Neurol Sci* 1997;24:29–36.

Lomen-Hoerth C, Murphy J, Langmore S, Kramer JH, Olney RK, Miller B. Are amyotrophic lateral sclerosis patients cognitively normal? *Neurology* 2003;60: 1094–1097.

Mier A. Respiratory muscle weakness. *Respir Med* 1990;84:351–359.

Newsom-Davis IC, Lyall RA, Leigh PN, et al. The effect of non-invasive positive pressure ventilation (NIPPV) on cognitive function in amyotrophic lateral sclerosis (ALS): a prospective study. *J Neurol Neurosurg Psychiatry* 2001;71: 482–487.

Przedborski S, Clarke PGH. Cell death pathways in amyotrophic lateral sclerosis. In Shaw P, Strong M (eds.). *Motor Neuron Disorders.* Philadelphia: Butterworth Heinemann; 2003, 357–377.

Ringholz GM, Appeal SH, Bradshaw M, et al. Prevalence and patterns of cognitive impairment in sporadic ALS. *Neurology* 2005;65:586–590.

Siobal M. The myth of hypoxic drive in chronic lung disease. Presentation at San Francisco General Hospital, Respiratory Care Services Forum: Selected Topics in Intensive Respiratory Care; April 13, 2007.

Strong M. ALS: One disease or many? *Amyotrophic Lateral Sclerosis* 2007; 8(Suppl 1):7–8.

Strong M, Rosenfeld J. Amyotrophic lateral sclerosis: a review of current concepts. *ALS Other Motor Neuron Disord* 2003;4:136–143.

Strong MJ, Grace GM, Orange JB, et al. A prospective study of cognitive impairment in ALS. *Neurology* 1999;53:1665–1670.

Strong M, Lomen-Hoerth C, Wenchang Y. Cognitive impairment in the motor neuron disorders. In Shaw P, Strong M (eds.). *Motor Neuron Disorders.* Philadelphia: Butterworth Heinemann; 2003, pp. 145–166.

Wilson CM, Grace GM, Munoz DG, et al. Cognitive impairment in sporadic ALS: a pathologic continuum underlying a multisystem disorder. *Neurology* 2001;57: 651–657.

Woolley S, Katz JS. Cognitive and Behavioral Impairment in ALS. *Phy Med Rehabil Clin N Am* 2008;19:607–617.

QUESTIONS FOR RESEARCH

In motor neuron disease, a patient's responses to weakening respiratory muscles are individualized. A patient's subjective and physiological reaction to diaphragmatic muscle weakness varies and is of interest to RCPs, physicians, nurses, physical therapists, and others who care for this population.

1. What factors contribute to an individual's *ability* to use accessory muscles to generate normal vital capacity in the face of chronic diaphragmatic weakness?

2. What factors contribute to one's ability to compensate for chronic respiratory insufficiency (elevated PCO_2, normal pH, elevated HCO_3^-) *without significant dyspnea*?

3. How does cognitive impairment or FTD affect a patient's ability to comply with noninvasive ventilation?

4. How much of an effect does respiratory insufficiency have on cognitive impairment, and how much of this impairment is reversible with intervention?

The Upper Airway

CHAPTER OUTLINE

CASE HISTORY

Mr. Miller, a 53-year-old man, was a cellist in a large urban symphony. He and his wife had no children of their own, but he volunteered as a teacher in a youth orchestra for low-income children. He was an avid golfer and tennis player and prided himself in being more than competent in both. He and his wife participated in regional tennis competitions. He had a family history of hypercholesteremia, for which he was prescribed statins. His only other medication was baby aspirin. His blood pressure was normal. His only hospitalization had been for arthroscopic surgery for meniscus repair of the right knee.

Mr. Miller began to have choking spells while drinking cold liquids and noted that his voice was more "gravely." After developing dyspnea at night because of accumulation of saliva in the back of this throat, he sought care from his primary care physician. His physician noted atrophy and fasciculations of the tongue and suspected amyotrophic lateral sclerosis (ALS). He was referred to a speech language pathologist for a barium swallow. Although no aspiration was noted, there was mild retention of barium and dribbling into the vallecula epiglottica.

Mr. Miller sought a second opinion from a neurologist. The neurologist noted Mr. Miller's general physical examination as unremarkable—weight, 165 pounds; blood pressure, 118/80; pulse, 70; and respirations, 12. Forced vital capacity (FVC) was 95% of predicted. There were no contractures or trophic changes in the skin. Motor and sensory functions were normal. Sternocleidomastoids were strong bilaterally. Muscle strength was normal throughout, as was muscle mass.

Mr. Miller, as usual, was cooperative and charming. He was fully oriented to time, place, and person. Recent and remote memory was intact. Simple calculations were done without difficulty.

After examination of innervation of the seventh cranial nerve, however, the neurologist noted that the tongue was weak, as Mr. Miller was unable to protrude the cheek with his tongue. Rapid movements of the tongue were markedly slowed. His speech was slow and slurred, but comprehensible. His gag was hyperactive. EMG studies were ordered and further confirmed a diagnosis of motor neuron disease. He was referred to an ALS clinic for follow-up.

When seen in the ALS clinic for his second visit 4 months later, Mr. Miller reported increased difficulty swallowing. He said that his saliva was thick and stringy and difficult to manage during the day, but thin and watery at night, causing more frequent bouts of choking. Most disconcerting was that Mr. Miller had begun to have episodes in which he felt that his throat had completely closed and that he could not breathe. These episodes resolved spontaneously, and he could not identify a trigger. He also reported that he could not blow his nose and that his nose dripped and saliva drooled from his mouth—the combination was embarrassing and distressing. He also reported he could no longer "bear down" during a bowel movement and worried about his risk of fecal impaction.

Mr. Miller had lost 15 pounds unintentionally. Eating had become more difficult. He found thick shakes to be the easiest to swallow without choking. A percutaneous endoscopic gastrostomy tube placement was recommended, but he declined. Amitriptyline was prescribed to treat sialorrhea. Help from the speech language pathologist was suggested to reduce laryngospasm. The clinic dietitian suggested ways of increasing calories.

Although his dysarthria and dysphagia continued to worsen, Mr. Miller continued with his golf and tennis. Drooling made performing with the symphony difficult. He resorted to placing paper towels in the roof of his mouth to absorb the saliva that he was no longer able to manage, changing them frequently. He eventually took a leave of absence from the symphony, but continued his volunteer work with the youth orchestra.

A year later Mr. Miller reported little change in his golfing or tennis games, although he said ruefully that they had not improved. He admitted that his stamina had diminished, and now he used a cart instead of walking the golf course. The clinic respiratory care practitioner (RCP) reported that his FVC values had not unchanged. Fine motor coordination was diminished in one hand. He was having difficulty buttoning his shirts. Speech had become unintelligible. Communication was accomplished using a LiteWriter, which vocalized his typewritten words. Sialorrhea remained his primary complaint. Robinul and Sal-tropine (oral Atropine) had been tried without success. He reported sleeping well but used a wedge to increase the head of his bed to avoid aspiration and choking. Laryngospasms continued, especially at night.

At year 3, Mr. Miller's FVC had decreased to 85% of predicted. Hand weakness continued, and there was generalized weakness in his limbs, most noticeably the biceps and triceps. There was no tongue movement. Swallowing had worsened, and maintaining weight was difficult. A percutaneous endoscopic gastrostomy was again refused. Botox injections were recommended to treat his refractory sialorrhea.

Six months later, Mr. Miller was again seen in the ALS clinic. He now reported very low energy and admitted dyspnea with activities. He reported sleeping in his recliner to avoid choking on saliva, which had not abated. He declined use of an electric hospital bed. The RCP was unable to obtain pulmonary function tests because of loss of oropharyngeal muscle tone. Noninvasive positive pressure ventilation (NPPV) was trialed in clinic, but Mr. Miller found it uncomfortable and declined its use. The RCP instructed Mr. Miller in manual chest hyperinflation with a resuscitation bag and mask. He was also instructed in self-Heimlich, and his wife in "quad" coughing technique. Profuse sialorrhea remained his primary issue, although his extremities continued to lose strength. Energy conservation was discussed, and specific suggestions were made. His wife stated that he was easily frustrated at no longer being able to play golf and tennis and perform routine daily activities, such as bathing and dressing himself because of arm and hand weakness.

On his last clinic visit, Mr. Miller had increasing limb weakness. His gait was unsteady, with his endurance limited to walking two blocks. His wife reported recent falls at home. A walker had been ordered on a previous visit. A lightweight power wheelchair was ordered on this visit. Increased dyspnea and daytime fatigue were reported. Repeated Botox injections had improved sialorrhea slightly, but this had led to increased oral bacteria. Techniques for improving oral hygiene were discussed. Mr. Miller and his wife discussed his end-of-life wishes. He elected to sign an advanced directive specifying no intubation or resuscitation. He decided to enter hospice care with the help and support of his family, neurologist, and multidisciplinary clinic staff.

INTRODUCTION TO THE UPPER AIRWAY

Bulbar muscles control speech and swallowing. Bulbar muscle weakness, as evidenced by slurring of speech, reduced speech rate, hoarse voice, and change in tone or pitch, is the first symptom of ALS in approximately 20% of patients. Dysarthria (spasticity or weakness of the muscles of speech) is observed more commonly than dysphagia (difficulty with eating) as the initial bulbar symptom. Early signs of bulbar muscle weakness include a change in vocal quality, hypernasality, and changes in speech with fatigue (Ball et al., 2001). Symptom management for dysarthria includes palatal lifts to treat hypernasality, vocal fold augmentation procedures, or Botox injections to improve voice quality, and assistive devices to improve communication.

Early symptoms of dysphagia include difficulty chewing, increased length of time to complete meals, and increased number of choking episodes (Rowland, 2003). Denervation of muscles of the upper airway puts patients at risk for aspiration of saliva, gastric contents, and food or thin liquids. In ALS, dysphagia management focuses primarily on nutrition and increasing caloric intake in the face of swallowing difficulties. Aspiration avoidance is one component of improving nutritional status.

ANATOMY AND PHYSIOLOGY

Early anatomists thought the lower brain stem resembled a flower bulb, resulting in the name bulbar. Neuronal traffic passes through the brainstem. The lowermost cranial nerves supply muscles of the oropharynx (tongue and palate). It is difficult to distinguish between pure upper motor neuron (UMN) and lower motor neuron (LMN) involvement on the bulbar muscles. All of the articulators (tongue, lips, palate) can be affected by UMN or LMN weakness; however, neurologic evaluation of the face and oropharynx reveal the following signs often attributed to the upper and lower neurons:

- UMN impairment affects the tongue, lips, facial muscles, and palate.
  Clinical signs include spasticity of the vocal folds, tightness, slurred speech and slowed tongue movement, exaggerated pharyngeal reflex, and spasticity of the vocal folds.
- LMN impairment affects the tongue, lips, facial muscles, and palate.
  Clinical signs include fasciculations of the tongue, pharynx and facial muscles, muscle atrophy, weakness, depressed or absent pharyngeal reflex, and vocal cord weakness evidenced by reduced abduction or adduction of the true vocal folds.

STRUCTURES OF THE UPPER AIRWAY

The University of Washington Neuromuscular Clinic for Swallowing and Speech Disorders is a multidisciplinary clinic that includes otolaryngology/head and neck surgery, speech pathology, neurologic nursing, and dietetics with consultation from pulmonary medicine, gastroenterology, and neurology. They have managed the care of hundreds of ALS patients. Their systematic review of the mouth and upper airway is summarized later here and is instructive for RCPs and others whose focus is typically the lower airway and muscles of respiration (Hillel & Miller, 1989).

Physical findings of bulbar ALS are divided into four muscle groups: tongue and lips; palate and muscles of mastication; neck, shoulders, trapezius, and vocal cords; and diaphragm, intercostals and accessory muscles of respiration.

The Tongue

A slowed speech rate is frequently an early sign of UMN involvement. When a patient cannot move the tongue beyond the lips, speech becomes impaired, and intelligibility is reduced. Speech rate is slowed, and consonants are slurred. When the tongue cannot be moved beyond the incisors (the cutting teeth), changes in food consistency (very soft food and thickened liquids) are necessary to reduce chances of aspiration. A common test is to have the patient use the tongue to push through the cheek against the examiner's finger. The inability to do so is a sign of difficulty with the oral transport phase of swallowing.

The Lips

Lip weakness will progressively lead to food spillage, impaired speech, and drooling. Lip strength is tested by having the patient hold a seal while puffing out the cheeks or suck on a clinician's gloved finger. Lip weakness will impair a patient's ability to maintain a tight seal around a mouthpiece when performing pulmonary function testing. Clinicians will need to use an oronasal mask for testing when this occurs. An inability to generate a lip seal and mandible muscle weakness will also inform clinician's choice of interface with NPPV.

The Palate

A speech language pathologist will examine the gag reflex to see whether the palate is able to elevate completely. Palatal dysfunction results in a hypernasal quality to speech. It is an early symptom in bulbar onset ALS (Yorkston et al., 1993). As palatal dysfunction advances, there is increased communication between the oral and nasal pharynx. A loss of closure of the veil between the soft palate and posterior nasopharyngeal wall (velum) can result in nasal regurgitation. Patients will not be able to use a straw. Palatal weakness can be assessed by having the patient blow out the cheeks while checking for air escaping from the nose.

Muscles of Mastication

Weakness in the muscles of mastication (chewing) results in the jaw being pulled down by gravity. This leaves the mouth open. Air no longer flows through the nose, whose purpose is to warm, humidify, and filter inspired air. Mouth breathing results in dry lips and mouth and tenacious oral secretions. Hydrating mouthwashes and oral gels may alleviate these symptoms to some degree. Good oral hygiene is essential to reduce the risk of aspirating residual food particles or aspirating oral bacteria, which can cause pneumonia.

Muscles of Swallowing

Swallowing is a complex process that appears to involve both UMNs and LMNs. It originates in the medulla and involves both voluntary and reflexive mechanisms. There are four phases: oral preparation, oral, pharyngeal, and esophageal. Dysfunction in any phase can limit food intake, contribute to choking, or increase aspiration risk.

This is the swallowing sequence:

1. The lips close. The jaws provide mastication, and the tongue moves food within the mouth.
2. The tongue moves food into a ball (bolus) in preparation for swallowing.
3. The velum (nasopharyngeal port) closes to prevent nasal regurgitation.
4. The tongue moves the bolus to the pharynx.
5. The larynx closes and moves up and out opening the upper esophageal sphincter.
6. The muscle of the tongue and lateral pharyngeal walls, with minimal contribution, if any, of the posterior pharyngeal wall squeezes the bolus into the esophagus.
7. The esophageal sphincter opens, and food is moved down the esophagus in waves.

The Sternocleidomastoid and Trapezius Muscles

Weakness in the sternocleidomastoid and trapezius muscles, which RCPs usually think of as accessory muscles of inspiration, results in the inability to keep the head from falling backward and the inability to raise the arms. This impacts oral intake in two ways. First, an inability to raise the arms will impair a patient's ability to feed himself or herself, cut food, and prepare meals. Second, having the head fall backward during swallowing increases the risk of aspiration. Patients are encouraged to use a chin tuck position during swallowing. The head-down position tucks the inlet to the larynx under the tongue base. In this position, food and liquid will be directed into the esophagus and not into the trachea, which lies directly posterior to it. Patients with limited hyolaryngeal elevation are encouraged to keep the chin in a neutral position to avoid aspiration. Mobile arm supports and braces can better allow a patient to eat independently.

Vocal Cords

The upper and lower respiratory tracts are anatomically divided by the vocal cords. Vocal cords insert on the posterior surface of the thyroid cartilage and project from the paired arytenoid cartilages. Vocal cords open and close to allow for vocalization. Vibration resulting from air moving through the vocal cords creates sound. Cord tension determines the pitch. The intensity of sound is determined by the volume of air flowing through the cords. In ALS, arytenoid abduction (movement away from midline) and adduction (movement toward median line) may be impaired. Patients may lose function in one or both vocal folds. A loss of vocal cord function reduces the flow of air necessary for speech. Vocal cords also must be able to close sufficiently to allow intrathoracic pressure to build, allowing the high velocity of air to flow through the cords during a cough. Collagen injections have been used to improve vocal cord closure.

Muscles of Respiration

The muscles of respiration are innervated by the third, fourth, and fifth cervical nerve segments. These nerves supply the diaphragm and, along with the thoracic nerves, the intercostal muscles. The muscles of respiration are the primary site of the onset of ALS in less than 2% of cases; however, denervation of respiratory muscles will occur eventually and is often the cause of death.

Respiratory muscle strength is inferred predominantly from measures of FVC, maximum inspiratory pressure, and peak cough flow. These measures are difficult to obtain in patients with moderate-to-severe bulbar muscle involvement caused by poor glottic and oropharyngeal muscle tone. Sniff negative inspiratory pressure may be used with greater success in these patients to test for diaphragmatic muscle strength.

CLINICAL IMPLICATIONS OF IMPAIRED UPPER AIRWAY

Airway Obstruction

Spasticity and weakness in the tongue and soft palate may lead to physical obstruction. During sleep in the supine position, the base of the tongue can fall posteriorly, creating a partial blockage or complete obstruction of the upper airway. Patients with moderate to severe bulbar muscle impairment may experience pharyngeal collapse on inhalation. This has implications for obtaining accurate and meaningful results during pulmonary function testing.

Sialorrhea

Bulbar muscle weakness results in impaired secretion clearance and an inability to manage saliva (sialorrhea). Although patients do not produce excessive saliva, tongue spasticity and weakness lead to an inability to coordinate saliva. Weakness of the swallowing muscles limits clearance of saliva. This facilitates drooling or coughing and choking on saliva.

Laryngospasm

Laryngospasm, the reflexive tightening or complete closure of the larynx, may also occur in patients with bulbar muscle involvement. It can be a terrifying experience, as it can occur suddenly, and patients feel unable to breathe. Triggers vary, and patients should make note of what situations appear to stimulate laryngoconstriction. Patients should be assured that laryngospasms are not life threatening and will resolve spontaneously after less than 60 seconds.

Aspiration Pneumonia

Denervation of muscles of the upper respiratory tract put ALS patients at risk of lower-airway contamination, aspiration pneumonia, or pneumonitis. Aspiration is usually of three types:

- Bacteria from a colonized oropharynx entering the lung
- Gastric acid entering the lung

- Water, food particles, or other inert substances entering the lung

The lower respiratory tract is a sterile field, and the healthy functioning of the upper respiratory tract serves to maintain this sterility. Cough and the mucociliary escalator provide defenses against bacteria contaminating the lower airway. Impairment of these protective mechanisms puts patients at risk of lower-airway infections. Advanced age, disruption of normal oral flora by medication, serious illness, and malnutrition also impair one's natural defenses against pneumonia.

In healthy individuals, the oropharynx is colonized by both aerobic and anaerobic organisms. Normal oral flora inhibits the growth of pathogens; however, it is not uncommon for individuals with neurologic diseases and malnutrition to have oropharyngeal colonization by enteric gram-negative bacilli. The more serious an illness, the greater the chances of gram-negative colonization (Niederman, 1990). Aspiration may be observed or silent. Aspiration of contaminated oropharyngeal secretions is the primary cause of most pneumonia. Pneumonia is the third most common reason for hospitalization in ALS, after acute respiratory failure and complications of malnutrition (Lechtzin et al., 2001).

Patients and their families should be told to contact their health care providers at the earliest signs of fever, chills, and productive cough. Debilitated patients with weakened muscles of respiration will have to be monitored closely to avoid respiratory failure.

Oral Hygiene

In a related vein, patients with flail arms and loss of hand strength have difficulty maintaining good oral hygiene. Caregivers will need to assist with tooth brushing and flossing. Assistive devices may be useful. An electric toothbrush has a large handle for easier grip and eliminates the need for up and down movement. A portable suction unit with an oral wand aids in rinsing the mouth if aspiration is feared. Professional cleaning and evaluation of gums and teeth are important to avoid or treat caries and unhealthy bacteria. Overgrowth of infectious oral flora combined with an inability to protect the lower airway fully from oropharyngeal secretions puts a patient at risk of aspiration pneumonia. Halitosis should alert clinicians to this possibility and prompt discussion of importance of oral hygiene and ways to maintain it.

Involuntary Emotional Expression

Prominent bulbar involvement is associated with involuntary emotional expressive disorder (IEED), commonly known as psuedobulbar affect. This may manifest as uncontrolled, exaggerated, or inappropriate laughing or crying. It may also be seen in uncharacteristic frustration, anger, or irritability. IEED presents a challenge for clinicians attempting to obtain patient cooperation in pulmonary function testing, lung hyperinflation, or cough maneuver training. It also can create embarrassment for patients and frustration at being unable to express their true emotions.

The frontal and temporal cortices control mood and emotional expression. It is hypothesized that a loss of cortical neurons and disruption of the corticobulbar tract results in IEED. A similar pathology may result in frontotemporal dementia. Apathy, impaired judgment, and a lack of insight into the dire implications of ALS are common features of frontotemporal dementia. Cognitive impairment in ALS is covered in greater detail in Chapter 2.

ASSESSMENT TECHNIQUES

ALS Functional Rating Score

Speech language pathologists score the degree of bulbar muscle impairment using the ALSFRS-R bulbar subscore. Speech, salivation, and swallowing are rated on a scale of 4 to 0, with 4 denoting normal processes and 0 loss of abilities. As symptoms progress, patients will move from normal speech to "intelligible with repeating" and then "speech combined with augmentative and alternative communication," and finally, "loss of useful speech" and complete reliance on alternative communication. Patients will also move from normal swallowing and eating habits to occasional choking, after which changes in dietary consistency will be necessary. As severity progresses, patients will need to supplement their oral intake with tube feedings. Eventually they will not be able to take any food or liquid by mouth, relying exclusively on parenteral or enteral feedings.

Intelligibility and Rate of Speech

Speech language pathologists use a variety of strategies to objectively measure progression of speech and swallowing impairment. Intelligibility can be measured with the Sentence Intelligibility Test in which patients are asked to read a series of 11 sentences of increasing length, from 5 to 15 words. The test is timed and speech rated for intelligibility and rate in words per minute. In their study of early bulbar signs in ALS, Ball et al. (2001) found the decline in speaking rate to be an early bulbar symptom while intelligibility remained stable. In researching sensitive predictors of early bulbar involvement, they found that tongue movement and cough force showed a linear decline at the speaking rate of 150 words per minute. Clinicians should remain patient when communicating with those who have bulbar involvement. Patients often report intense frustration when the "mouth no longer works as fast as their brain."

Swallowing Evaluations

Silent aspiration can lead to pneumonia, one cause of acute respiratory failure, emergency intubation, and ventilation in ALS patients. When laryngeal dysfunction is suspected and evaluated in the clinic, a swallowing evaluation will confirm the presence of aspiration so that steps to avoid it can be discussed with the patient. When chewing and swallowing difficulties are noted, swallowing evaluations are conducted, and techniques to improve oral nutrition are recommended.

Swallowing function in myasthenia gravis, an autoimmune disorder of the neuromuscular junction with the common symptom of bulbar muscle involvement, has informed the evaluation of silent aspiration in ALS (Higo et al., 2005). Normally, upward movement of the larynx tilts the epiglottis, causing closure of the laryngeal opening and protecting the airway. Impaired laryngeal elevation is correlated with aspiration. The Repetitive Saliva Swallowing Test can be used to screen for aspiration in patients with dysphagia. With one hand on the patient's larynx, the patient is asked to dry swallow as many times as he or she can in 30 seconds. The larynx will elevate with each swallow and is counted. If a patient can swallow only one or two times in 30 seconds, he or she is at risk for aspiration. This simple test may be used as a screen for more conclusive assessments using videofluoroscopy or Fiberoptic Endoscopic Evaluation of Swallowing, the "gold standards" of swallowing evaluations.

In videofluoroscopy the patient swallows a bolus with contrast medium. The bolus is then followed radiographically as it moves from mouth to pharynx through the upper esophageal sphincter. The patient is assessed for bolus holding in the oral cavity, velopharyngeal seal, tongue base movement, pharyngeal constriction, laryngeal elevation, upper esophageal sphincter opening, response to pharyngeal residue, and aspiration.

Fiberoptic Endoscopic Evaluation of Swallowing can be performed in the outpatient clinic setting and does not involve radiation. Using a flexible endoscope direct visualization of laryngeal function, secretion management, and observation of natural eating and drinking behavior can be observed over a long period of time. Swallowing evaluations focus on patient education and strategies to make chewing and swallowing easier and more comfortable while reducing aspiration risk. These strategies may include holding the bolus in the mouth a few seconds before swallowing, holding the breath (closing the larynx intentionally), tucking the chin, taking smaller bites or sips, or washing food down with liquids. Education provided during these tests improves oral nutrition and reduces loss of muscle mass caused by malnutrition in patients able and willing to follow speech language pathologist recommendations.

SYMPTOM MANAGEMENT

Sialorrhea

The prevalence of clinically significant drooling in ALS is estimated at 50% (Jackson et al., 2007). Saliva volume is estimated to be 0.5 to 2 quarts per day. Saliva is produced by three glands: submandibular (approximately 70% of the volume), parotid (25%), and sublingual (5%). Consistency of saliva varies by gland: Submandibular glands produce predominantly serous saliva that has mucoid qualities. Parotid produces serous saliva, and sublingual glands secrete both mucoid and serous saliva.

An inability to manage saliva negatively impacts patients' quality of life and puts them at risk for aspiration of oral secretions and resulting bacterial pneumonia. Drooling is embarrassing for many patients and increases caregiver burden because of the need for frequent oral suctioning and tissue changes.

The most common treatments for sialorrhea are anticholinergic medications. These include the short-acting agents hyoscyamine sulfate (Levsin), glycopyrrolate (Robinul), and oral atropine, sublingual liquid or tablets. Longer acting agents include amitriptyline (Elavil), nortriptyline (Pamelor), transdermal scopolamine, and diphenydramine (Benadryl). Botulinum toxin (Botox) injections into the parotid or sub-mandibular glands are safe and effective for treating sialorrhea when patients do not respond to anticholinergic medications and have disabling sialorrhea (Giess et al., 2000). Two types of botulinum toxins have been researched in ALS, A and B (Verma & Steele, 2006; Costa et al, 2008). Botox B appears to be more effective that Botox A. Benefits of Botox injections can last for 8 to 12 weeks. When sialorrhea is not responsive to other treatments, low-dose radiation to the salivary glands is an option but is not frequently recommended by physicians.

Swallowing and Nutrition

Increased energy expenditure caused by respiratory insufficiency, weak-ened muscles, spasticity, and fasciculations as well as dysphagia contrib-utes to weight loss and dehydration. Impaired swallowing makes it difficult to increase caloric intake. Dehydration contributes to constipation. Speech language pathologists evaluate oropharyngeal dysfunction and make recommendations concerning diet and review strategies to maintain weight. The National Dysphagia Diet includes food texture and consis-tency guidelines. In multidisciplinary clinics. RCPs, SLPs, and dietitians work together to maintain respiratory and nutritional status.

Enteral Nutrition

Nutrition is an integral component of ALS care. If eating becomes bur-densome, meal times become significantly longer, or other nutritional strategies (such as liquid calorie supplements) are ineffective in preventing weight loss, tube feeding is recommended for a stable source of nutrition and hydration (Miller et al., 1999). Enteral nutrition may be a primary or supplemental form of meeting caloric requirements and providing hydration. It is also a route for medication administration. The best time to introduce enteral nutrition has not been established. A recent study showed some survival benefit if tube feeding is initiated before 10% of weight is lost from time of first clinic visit (Clavelou et al., 2007); however, there is little tolerance for *any* weight loss in ALS and every effort is made to maintain patients' weight.

As patients may see percutaneous endoscopic gastrostomy placement as a milestone in ALS decline, early discussion of risks and benefits with patients and family members is useful (Desport et al., 2005). With the use of percutaneous endoscopic gastrostomy and the resulting increase in protein and calorie intake, weight stabilization or modest weight gain has been demonstrated (Mitsumoto et al., 2003). This is preferable to trying to gain back weight after a large amount has been lost. The risk of post-operative complications after percutaneous endoscopic gastrostomy increases when the FVC falls below 50% of predicted (Kasarskis et al., 1999). Mortality and morbidity after this procedure are often caused by diaphragm splinting and respiratory insufficiency (Mathus-Vliegen et al., 1994). This is another reason for early discussion of enteral nutrition.

Tracheostomy

For patients with severe bulbar dysfunction for whom sialorrhea is poorly controlled, bypassing the upper airway and allowing spontaneous ventilation via tracheostomy tube are options. Patients whose muscles of respiration remain functional and are able to maintain ventilation and oxygenation may consider this option. A tracheostomy aspiration suction tube, designed for patients who require placement of a tracheostomy tube due to dysphagia, may provide an effective means of managing aspiration. The tracheostomy aspiration suction tube collects and drains aspirated material, which pools above the inflated balloon-like cuff, keeping it from entering the lower airway.

NPPV delivered via nasal or oronasal mask is generally poorly tolerated by patients with severe bulbar symptoms. Assisted ventilation via tracheostomy is usually considered a life support measure; however, in this instance, if it is used intermittently to manage nocturnal hypoventilation and to rest muscles of respiration for brief periods during the day, it may improve quality of life and remains within the arena of palliative care.

COMMUNICATION AUGMENTATION FOR PATIENTS

Speech language pathologists with a specialty in augmentative and alternative communication greatly improve the quality of life of patients with ALS. Communication augmentation can be as simple as alphabet boards, voice amplifiers, and type-and-talk devices and as sophisticated as computer-based speech generating devices and eye gaze systems (Murphy,

2004). Brain–computer interfaces and thought translation devices are new communication methods. Prosthetic devices, such as palatal lift or palatal augmentation prostheses, can reduce hypernasality and improve articulation (Andersen et al., 2005).

Call chimes are an important means of communicating with household members who need to be summoned for assistance. Call chimes can be adapted for hand and arm weakness and the loss of fine motor skills. Energy conservation is emphasized as all muscle groups weaken. Using a voice amplifier, even when speech is intelligible, reduces the need to project the voice in order to be heard.

COMMUNICATION TECHNIQUES FOR CAREGIVERS AND MEDICAL PERSONNEL

Increased age is the major risk factor for the sporadic form of ALS with the highest incidence rate in the 60- to 69-year age group (Armon, 2003). At this age, normal decline in hearing, eyesight, and speech is common. When communicating with patients with speech impairment, we may be so focused on understanding the words and deciphering their meaning that we forget that we might not be heard and understood by our aging patients. Here are tips for communicating with people with sensory losses (Guion, 2007).

Eyesight

A loss of elasticity in the lens of the eye, increased density, rigidity, and flattening of the convexity of the cornea cause vision to decline by the age of 40 years, and by the age of 70 years, poor vision is commonplace. A loss of elasticity in the iris, decreased size of the pupil, and increased opacity of the lens combine to reduce the amount of light entering the eye and increase the sensitivity to glare. Lens rigidity diminishes visual acuity so that words may appear blurred and images muted.

To mitigate these age-related visual losses, practitioners can make simple accommodations that will greatly improve communication. Do not stand in front of a window or bright light source. This will cause you to be "back lit" and will make visual cues of communication (mouth and facial expressions) difficult to see. Printed materials should be in larger type sizes and in contrasting colors.

Hearing

Thinning and fibrosis of the tympanic membrane leads to age-related hearing loss. High-pitched frequencies are difficult to distinguish. Degenerative changes in cochlea, auditory nerve pathways, and cilia decrease the ability to distinguish between consonants. Lowering one's voice and speaking slowly and distinctly will improve your ability to be understood and the patient's retention of information. Face the patient when speaking, as lip reading can augment listening to words. Do not cover the mouth during speech, and do not chew gum during conversation.

SUMMARY

As a result of their negative impact on social interaction, bulbar symptoms can be extremely distressing, can create frustration, and may lead to social isolation. Difficulty swallowing and masticating changes eating from an enjoyable experience to one of sheer survival. A meal that once took 15 to 30 minutes to consume may take over an hour, contributing to exhaustion. Meals shared with friends and family, especially during holiday celebrations, may become fraught with anxiety because of self-consciousness and fear of choking. The experience of fully enjoying new foods and discovering new restaurants is altered forever; however, nutrition can be maintained. Aspiration risks can be reduced. Speech can be augmented throughout the course of the disease process.

Evidence-based guidelines are available and assessment by a speech language pathologist is essential. A thorough understanding of the role and function of the upper and lower airways can guide symptom management. If patients and their care providers think creatively and behave proactively, quality of life can be maintained to the degree defined by the person with ALS.

REFERENCES

Andersen, P, Borasio G, Dengler R, et al. EFNS task force on management of amyotrophic lateral sclerosis: guidelines for diagnosing and clinical care of patients and relatives. *Eur J Neurol* 2005;12:921–938.

Armon C. Epidemiology of amyotrophic lateral sclerosis/motor neuron disease. In Shaw P, Strong M (eds.). *Motor Neuron Disorders*. Philadelphia: Butterworth Heinemann of Elsevier's Health Sciences, 2003, pp. 167–206.

Ball L, Willis A, Beukelman DR, Pattee GL. A protocol for identification of early bulbar signs in amyotrophic lateral sclerosis. *J Neurol Sci* 2001;191:43–53.

Clavelou P, Ouchchane L, Gerbaud L, et al. Effects of tube-feeding on quality of life and survival in amyotrophic lateral sclerosis patients (a cohort study in 383 patients). *Amyotrophic Lateral Sclerosis* 2007;8(Suppl):68.

Costa J, Rocha ML, Ferreira J, et al. Botulinum toxin type-B improves sialorrhea and quality of life in bulbaronset amyotrophic lateral sclerosis. *J Neurol* 2008;255(4):545–550.

Desport JC, Mabrouk, T, Bouillet P, Perna A, Preux PM, Couratier P. Complications and survival following radiologically and endoscopically-guided gastrostomy in patients with amyotrophic lateral sclerosis. *Amyotrophic Lateral Sclerosis Other Motor Neuron Disord* 2005;6:88–93.

Giess R, Naumann M, Werner E, et al. Injections of botulinum toxin A into the salivary glands improve sialorrhea in amyotrophic lateral sclerosis. *J Neurol Neurosurg Psychiatry* 2000;69:121–123.

Guion L. Can you talk the talk (and be understood)? *AARC Times* 2007;31: 24–26.

Higo R, Nito T, Tayama N. Videofluoroscopic assessment of swallowing function in patients with myasthenia gravis. *J Neurol Sci* 2005;231:45–48.

Hillel A, Miller R. Bulbar amyotrophic lateral sclerosis: patterns of progression and clinical management. *Head Neck* 1989;January/February:51–59.

Jackson C, Gronseth G, Rosenfeld J, et al. A randomized, double-blind, palacebo-controlled study of the safety and efficacy of botulinum toxin type B (BTXB) for sialorrhea in ALS. *Amyotrophic Lateral Sclerosis* 2007;8(Suppl): 69–70.

Kasarskis EJ, Scarlata D, Hill R, Fuller C, Stambler N, Cedarbaum JM. A retrospective study of percutaneous endoscopic gastrostomy in ALS patients during the BDNF and CNTF trials. *J Neurol Sci* 1999;169:118–125.

Lechtzin N, Wiener CM, Clawson L, Chaudhry V, Diette GB. Hospitalization in amyotrophic lateral sclerosis: causes, costs, and outcomes. *Neurology* 2001;56: 753–757.

Mathus-Vliegen LMH, Louwerse LS, Merkus MP, et al. Percutaneous endoscopic gastrostomy in patients with amyotrophic lateral sclerosis and impaired pulmonary function. *Gastrointest Endosc* 1994;40:463–469.

Miller RG, Rosenberg JA, Gelinas DF, et al. Practice parameter: the care of the patient with amyotrophic lateral sclerosis (an evidence-based review): report of the Quality Standards Subcommittee of the American Academy of Neurology: ALS Practice Parameters Task Force. *Neurology* 1999;52:1311–1323.

Mitsumoto H, Davidson M, Moore D. ALS CARE Study Group. Percutaneous endoscopic gastrostomy (PEG) in patients with ALS and bulbar disfunction. *Amyotrophic Lateral Sclerosis Other Motor Neuron Disord* 2003;4:177–185.

Murphy J. Communication strategies of people with amyotrophic lateral sclerosis and their partners. *Amyotrophic Lateral Sclerosis Other Motor Neuron Dis* 2004; 5:121–126.

Niederman MS. Gram-negative colonization of the respiratory tract: pathogenesis and clinical consequences. *Semin Respir Infect* 1990;5:173–184.

Rowland LR. Clinical aspects of sporadic amyotrophic lateral sclerosis/motor neuron disease. In Shaw J, Strong M (eds.). *Blue Books of Practical Neurology: Motor Neuron Disorders.* Philadelphia: Butterworth & Heinemann; 2003, pp. 111–143.

Verma A, Steele J. Botulinum toxin improves sialorrhea and quality of life in bulbar amyotrophic lateral sclerosis. *Muscle Nerve* 2006;34(2):235–237.

Yorkston K, Strand E, Miller R, Hillel A, Smith K. Speech deterioration in amyotrophic lateral sclerosis: implications for timing of intervention. *J Med Speech-Language Pathol* 1993;1:35–46.

QUESTIONS FOR RESEARCH

1. In ALS patients with bulbar muscle weakness in need of noninvasive respiratory assistance, what pressures, flow rates, and inspiratory/expiratory ratios will increase acceptance and adherence to NPPV?

2. In ALS patients with severe bulbar weakness and poorly controlled sialorrhea, does tracheostomy significantly reduce aspiration and choking?

3. What are the most effective methods of managing symptoms of laryngospasm?

4. How can RCPs and SLPs work together to reduce aspiration risk and improve oral nutrition in ALS patients with bulbar muscle weakness?

The Lower Airway

CHAPTER OUTLINE

THE NORMAL LUNG

The normal lung is a sterile field and is free of bacteria below the larynx. The lower airway is composed of the conducting airways (trachea, bronchi, and nonrespiratory bronchioles) and respiratory units (respiratory bronchioles and alveoli). Oxygen and carbon dioxide are circulated through pulmonary vasculature that receives the entire cardiac output (Dantzker, 1995). Venous blood returns from the systemic tissues to the lungs for gas exchange. Knowledge of the form and function of the lower airway informs our ability to intervene in the management of pulmonary complications in amyotrophic lateral sclerosis (ALS). Detailed descriptions of the functional anatomy of the respiratory system can be found in most respiratory therapy textbooks. Later here is a brief review of the lower airway and its primary functions.

LARYNX—THE DIVIDING LINE

Definition

The larynx is the organ of voice production. It is the valve that divides the upper and the lower airway, sitting between the pharynx and the trachea.

Composition

The larynx is composed of connective tissue, ligaments, and elastic membranes housed within a bony structure, the cricothyroid joint. The thyroid cartilage rotates on the cricothyroid joint, allowing for lengthening of the vocal folds. Innervation of the motor nerves of the larynx and upper airway comes from cranial nerves V, VII, IX, X, and XII and cervical nerves 1 to 3 (Dantzker, 1995). Muscles that surround the larynx allow for movement forward and backward and up and down.

Function

The larynx participates in three main functions: speech, swallowing, and coughing.

Speech is made possible by the position and tension of the vocal folds. The adduction (moving toward midline) and abduction (moving away from midline) of the vocal folds control air movement from the trachea to the pharynx. The role of the larynx in *swallowing* is primarily to direct food away from the trachea by moving it instead into the adjacent esophagus. The epiglottis, which sits at the base of the tongue, is an elastic flap that covers the opening to the larynx during swallowing. Simultaneous adduction of the vocal folds, upward movement of muscles surrounding the larynx, and backward and downward movement of the epiglottis combine to propel solids and liquids from the mouth toward the opening of the stomach.

Coughing is the primary defense against particles and mucus that collect in the larger airways. It also protects the lower airway from food and other particles if the epiglottis is poorly functioning and unable to guard fully against aspiration. The essential role of coughing in ALS will receive a more detailed description later in this chapter.

An additional function of the larynx is its role in increasing intrathoracic and intra-abdominal pressure. Adduction of the vocal folds allows for pressure to build within the lungs after hyperexpansion. This increased pressure allows for the expulsive airflow after vocal cord abduction that defines an effective cough. Intra-abdominal pressure allows for effective vomiting, urination, and defecation.

Denervation of laryngeal nerves disrupts all of the functions of the larynx. One or both vocal folds may lose innervation. In ALS, this process is gradual. As covered in the previous chapter on the upper airway, neurologists, speech language pathologists, and respiratory care practitioners (RCPs) work together to identify laryngeal muscle weakness. When it occurs, patients and family members need education tools to augment speech and guard against aspiration and secretion retention. These tools are covered in detail in Chapter 7.

CONDUCTING AIRWAYS

Definition

The conducting airways direct oxygen-enriched air from the nose and mouth to alveolar sacs where it diffuses across the alveolar–capillary membrane and into the pulmonary vessels.

The trachea, right and left main stem bronchi, and nonrespiratory bronchioles make up the conducting airways. The trachea begins just below the larynx and is composed of U-shaped cartilaginous rings that resist collapse under high intrathoracic pressures. It sits anterior to the esophagus. The close proximity of trachea and esophagus increases the risk of aspirating material from the upper airway when the vocal cords and epiglottis are compromised.

The right main stem bronchus, larger and less deviated at the bifurcation than the left, branches from the trachea. Its direct extension from the trachea explains the more frequent aspiration of foreign material into the right lung (Carden et al., 2005). The airways continue branching until they reach the terminal bronchioles.

Composition

The bronchial walls are composed of epithelial cells, columnar cells, basal cells, brush cells, and goblet cells. Below the epithelial cells lie the basement membrane, submucosal glands, and smooth muscle. Above lay the cilia, tiny hair-like structures bathed in the thin liquid sol layer. Finally, a gel layer with its viscoelastic lining compels mucus upward toward the trachea by the rhythmic beating of the cilia. Mucus must have the correct balance of viscosity and elasticity to interact optimally with the cilia and promote mucociliary clearance (Rogers, 2007).

Bronchial secretions consist predominantly of mucus. Together, goblet cells, type II alveolar cells, serous cells, and Clara cells produce mucus. The latter two cells secrete anti-inflammatory, immunomodulatory, and antibacterial molecules, aiding in airway defense (Rogers, 2007). Mucus production is higher in the peripheral airways, and it is here that mucociliary transport is greatest. Mucus production is lower in the central airways where expiratory airflow is largely responsible for mucus transport (van der Schans, 2007).

Function

Bronchial epithelium is responsible for fluid and electrolyte balance within the airway and regulating sodium, potassium, and chloride ions. Glands within the bronchi contain serous cells that excrete water, ions and peptides, and goblet cells that excrete mucin. This serous lining is composed predominantly of water, greater than 90%. The viscous properties of mucus are due to glycoprotein, representing carbohydrate and protein molecules, and oligosaccharide side chains. These are the major components of the airway lining. Together they provide moisture and humidity to the conducting airways and form the mucus escalator blanket responsible for moving foreign matter and infectious organisms from the lungs.

RESPIRATORY UNITS

Definition

Respiration refers to gas exchange, the diffusion of oxygen and carbon dioxide across the alveolar-capillary membrane. Respiratory bronchioles, alveolar ducts, and alveolar sacs comprise the respiratory unit, also referred to as the pulmonary acinus because of their grape-like appearance. Below the terminal bronchioles, alveolar ducts line the airways, and the number of alveoli dramatically increases.

Composition

Each air sac incorporates a mesh of capillaries. A thin layer of surfactant reduces surface tension to keep alveoli patent. Alveolar epithelium regulates movement of fluids and substances across the alveolar-capillary membrane protecting the alveolus from fluid moving into or remaining in the sac (Carden et al., 2005). Alveoli are directly connected to one another through the *pores of Kohn*. These openings allow collateral circulation if peripheral airways become blocked. Allowing air to flow from well-ventilated lung segments to underventilated ones prevents or corrects atelectasis.

Function

After ventilation carries oxygen through the conducting airways, gaseous diffusion moves it through alveolar walls and into pulmonary vessels.

Pulmonary vasoconstriction in response to hypoxia shunts blood away from poorly ventilated alveoli. This response reduces ventilation–perfusion mismatch. Unfortunately, over time, chronic pulmonary vascular resistance can lead to right heart failure.

LOWER-AIRWAY DEFENSE SYSTEMS

Irritant Receptors

Chemical irritant receptors, found in the epithelial lining of the large airways, can be triggered by a variety of exogenous and endogenous stimuli. Exogenous stimuli such as cold air, allergens, smoke, fumes, or gases from the environment can stimulate a response, as can cellular inflammatory agents such as eosinophiles, neutrophiles, or paucigranulocytes from within the airway (King & Moores, 2008). Irritant receptors are found predominantly in the distal central airways and airway junctions (Boitano, 2006). They are also found in the nerves of the trachea and large bronchi. When irritant receptors are stimulated, cough, increased mucus production, and bronchoconstriction function to protect the airway.

Mucociliary Escalator

As the name implies, mucus and cilia work together to transport particles from the bronchioles to the oropharynx where they are removed by coughing, expectoration, or swallowing. The elastic mucus of the gel layer traps particles. The cilia, beating back and forth in their thin sol layer, move the trapped particles upward toward the oropharynx. The transportation rate of the mucociliary escalator is approximately 3 millimeters per minute, and 90% of particles deposited on the mucus layer are cleared in about 2 hours (Carden et al., 2005). In the absence of disease, bronchial secretions go unnoticed.

An ideal ratio of viscosity to elasticity is essential for mucociliary clearance (King & Rubin, 1994). During acute pulmonary infection, byproducts of inflammatory cells will increase viscosity. Changes in viscosity of the gel or sol layers will impair the airway cleansing mechanism. Inhalation of cigarette smoke, toxic fumes, and acute pulmonary infection will impair or paralyze cilia. Proteolytic enzymes impair mucus elasticity.

The lungs are self-cleaning and designed to maintain homeostasis. In the absence of underlying lung disease, patients with ALS should not produce more secretions nor have changes in mucus viscosity or elasticity;

however, decreased physical activity, dependence on wheelchair or bed rest, and chronic hypoventilation may reduce the lung's ability to propel healthy mucus upward.

Airflow velocity is determined by airway diameter plus airway pressure created by expiratory muscles. Airflow transport is greater in the central airways (van der Schans, 2007). Decreased airflow caused by respiratory muscle weakness may result in mucus secretion retention. Mucus pooling in the airways (stasis) can create a potential breeding ground for infection and puts patients with pulmonary muscle compromise at risk for respiratory failure.

Cough

Mechanism

Coughing is a common yet complex mechanism. It remains poorly understood, although its protective qualities are appreciated. It is a primary component of the lower-airway defense system. The necessary components of an effective cough are as follows:

- Isometric contraction of expiratory muscles
- Glottis closure
- Increased intrathoracic pressures
- Rapid glottis opening
- Expulsion of high velocity gas

Mucus is removed from the airway by the high velocity of expired gas across the mucus layer. Airway velocity increases through airway narrowing. During a forceful exhalation (cough), transmural pressure (pressure surrounding the airway) compresses and narrows the airway. Expiratory muscle or bulbar muscle weakness in ALS reduces airflow velocity and impedes mucus removal. In addition, an imbalance of thin serous and thicker mucoid secretions caused by dehydration or other factors may present a challenge to patients with weakened cough ability. Viscosity of mucus and patency of airway lumen are the primary factors affecting secretion removal.

Triggers

When patients present with a chronic cough, common causes should be considered and differentiated (Irwin et al., 2006). Obtaining the patient's medical history, employment history, reported triggers, and known allergens will assist clinicians in distinguishing among common etiologies. Pulmonary function studies may be useful to rule out flow restriction in response to lower-airway irritation. In ALS, three primary etiologies of cough should be considered: upper-airway cough syndrome, gastroesophageal reflux disease (GERD), and asthma or other eosinophilic syndrome.

Upper-Airway Cough Syndrome

Coughs caused by an upper-airway infection are primarily caused by rhinoviruses or seasonal allergic rhinitis. Allergic rhinitis, an inflammation of the nasal passages associated with thin nasal discharge and congestion, affects approximately 20% of people in the United States (Naclerio & Solomon, 1997). Sinus drainage into the posterior oropharynx (postnasal drip) causes irritation and the cough response. This is now referred to as upper-airway cough syndrome (Irwin et al., 2006). Chronic irritation and inflammation of the posterior oropharynx will continue to result in frequent, dry coughs until the virus runs it course or exposure to environmental allergens ceases.

GERD

GERD (gastroesophageal reflux disease) is common in the United States, affecting as much as 20% of the adult population (Manterola et al., 2002). GERD may occur in ALS as the result of diaphragmatic weakness involving the lower esophageal sphincter (Anneser & Borasio, 2003). It is hypothesized that gastric fluid regurgitation into the upper airway irritates the larynx, pharynx, and posterior nasal mucosa and has been linked to chronic sinusitis (Manterola et al., 2002). In a study of 230 patients, Manterola et al. found that subjects with symptomatic GERD and a positive pH study confirming a GERD diagnosis had significantly higher scores of upper-respiratory symptoms. GERD may be present in the absence of gastric discomfort and heartburn. GERD should be suspected if dry cough, serous sinus drainage, hoarseness, sore throat, or morning dry mouth is present and if treatment for these symptoms is unsuccessful. GERD and upper-airway cough syndrome often present with chronic cough but, in the absence of reactive airway disease, do not result in bronchoconstriction and airway obstruction.

Asthma

Asthma appears not to be a single disease but one of multiple, overlapping, and separate clinical syndromes. Allergic asthma symptoms can include wheezing, dyspnea, and cough that worsen at night, especially in the early morning hours if poorly controlled (King & Moores, 2008). The same triggers that cause sinusitis and upper-airway irritation (inhaled seasonal allergens, upper-respiratory infection) are suspected of provoking asthma symptoms (Corren, 2000). For treatment purposes, allergic rhinitis should be distinguished from infection. Pulmonary function tests will assist in differentiating asthma exacerbation from other diseases. One should suspect lower airway inflammation and bronchoconstriction if forced expiratory volume in 1 second is not proportional to forced vital capacity. A postbronchodilator percent-of-predicted forced expiratory volume in 1 second increase of 15% is diagnostic for asthma (King & Moores).

Significance in ALS

A chronic and persistent cough is annoying and disruptive to most people, but to people with ALS, it can be tiring to already weakened respiratory and abdominal muscles. Coughing disrupts sleep, interferes with eating, and contributes to fatigue. It can be frightening and generally reduces a patient's quality of life. Unless the patient has persistent bacterial bronchitis or bronchiectasis, secretion production is rarely a component of chronic cough (Irwin & Madison, 2000). If a definitive source of the cough can be identified, treatments can be prescribed. Examples include the following:

Allergic Rhinitis (Lee, 2008)

- Sinus irrigation (saline solution and sprays) used to remove allergens from nasal passages
- Second-generation antihistamines (e.g., loratadine, cetirizine, and desloratadine)
- Oral decongestants (phenylephrine, pseudoephedrine)
- Topical decongestants (oxymetazoline)
- Nasal corticosteroids (fluticasone, triamcinolone, mometasone, and budesonide)
- Inhaled antihistamine (azelastine)
- Immunotherapy (desensitization)

GERD (Anneser & Borasio, 2003)

- Antacids (calcium carbonate)
- H-2 receptor blockers (cimetidine, famotidine, nizatidine, and ranitidine)
- Proton pump inhibitors (omeprazole)

Asthma

- Inhaled corticosteroids: controller medications (beclomethasone, budesonide, flunisolide, fluticasone, mometasone, triamcinolone, and ciclesonide) (Sobande & Kercsmar, 2008)
- Inhaled beta agonists: rescue medications (short acting: metaproterenol, albuterol, pirbuterol, and levalbuterol) (Donahue, 2008)
- Inhaled beta agonists: controller medications (long acting: salmeterol, formoterol, arformoterol tartrate) (Donahue)
- Combination inhaled corticosteroids/beta agonists (budesonide/ formoterol and fluticasone/salmeterol) (Donahue)

Clinicians should consult the expert panel report of the National Institutes of Health's National Asthma Education and Prevention Program for detailed asthma management guidelines (2007).

In 2006, the American College of Chest Physicians published evidence-based clinical practice guidelines for the diagnosis and management of cough (Irwin et al., 2006). A thorough review of cough can be found in the *Acute and Chronic Cough in the Lung Biology in Health and Disease* series (Redington & Morice, 2005). It details the money spent on over-the-counter remedies and reviews currently available therapies. The authors note that the benefits of many cough treatments owe much of their success to the placebo effect, but this question remains: When is a cough a normal, airway protective response, and when is it abnormal and needs to be suppressed?

BRONCHIAL MUCUS

Airway secretions are the purview of pulmonologists and RCPs. Nurses and other allied health professionals seem happy to leave the role of mucus secretion assessment and removal to pulmonary clinical specialists. RCPs devote a great of their clinical practice to airway clearance techniques. RCPs who work with ALS and other neuromuscular diseases also focus on the twin goals of lung volume recruitment and airway secretion management. RCPs who treat patients in the outpatient setting take a proactive approach to respiratory care in hopes of avoiding hospital and emergency department admissions due to respiratory failure.

Few scientific data, however, are available to support many of the therapies used to treat suspected mucus secretion retention. To evaluate the current state of the art of mucus secretion, cough, and airway clearance, the American Association for Respiratory Care hosted the 39th *Respiratory Care* journal conference Airway Clearance: Physiology, Pharmacology, Techniques, and Practice. The speakers at the conference (respiratory therapists, physical therapists, basic scientists, epidemiologists, and pulmonary physicians) were challenged to find evidence to support or refute a number of "mucus myths" and reach consensus on their appropriateness to clinical practice (Rubin, 2007). Reports of conference proceedings were published in *Respiratory Care* in September and October of 2007.

To assist respiratory therapy students, RCPs, and others who work with people with ALS, the remainder of this chapter on the lower airway is devoted to a review of the physiology of mucus secretion production and pharmacologic interventions. Chapter 7 focuses on airway secretion management techniques.

Biophysiology of Airway Mucus Secretions

To put it very simply, acute airway mucus secretion is a good thing (airway protection and hydration), but too much (chronic hypersecretion) is bad, especially if combined with impaired clearance ability. Mucus lining the airway epithelium provides a barrier that inhibits bacterial growth and biofilm formation (Rubin, 2007). Its component cells have antibacterial and anti-inflammatory properties. The 12,000 liters of air inhaled each day include pollen, bacteria, mold, dust and, in urban areas, a host of other irritants (Rogers, 2007). In normal, healthy lungs, transitory mucus secretion and mucociliary clearance provide protection. Cough in response to inflammation, irritation, and impaired mucociliary clearance is also a normal healthy response.

The biophysical properties of mucus are largely determined by mucins, secretions containing mucopolysaccharides. Twenty human mucin genes (MUC) have been identified with two, MUC5AC and MUC5B, occurring in the normal respiratory tract. MUC5AC is generally expressed in goblet cells in the epithelium and is distributed in the tissue of the lung and nasopharynx. MUC5B is expressed in the seromucus glands of the submucosa and is distributed in the tissue of the lung, laryngeal submucosal glands, and nasopharynx. Once stimulated, for example, by a temporary inhaled irritant, mucin release from the cell is explosive, and expansive responding like a "jack-in-the-box" so not a moment is lost (Rogers, 2007). This is a normal and healthy response. In the small airways, where coughing is less effective, normal mucin response may put neuromuscular patients at risk for secretion retention and mucus plugging.

Mucolytics

Mucolytics are capable of dissolving or liquefying mucus. They accomplish this by chemically dividing water molecules within the disulfide bonds that link mucin monomers together, destroying the polymer chain, and thereby reducing secretion viscosity. N-acetyl L-cysteine (NAC), also written *N*-acetylcysteine, is the best known mucolytic. Aerosolized NAC was once used to treat exacerbations of chronic obstructive pulmonary disease (COPD), perhaps because of its success in reducing tracheobronchial secretion viscosity in vitro (Sheffner et al., 1964); however, a large, long-term, randomized, controlled study of NAC in COPD showed no clinical benefit, not improving pulmonary function, mucus clearance, or quality of life (Decramer et al., 2005). Clinical trials of aerosolized and oral NAC in chronic bronchitis have produced ambiguous data (Rogers, 2007). A meta-analysis of studies of mucolytic agents found that their use produced no significant improvements in pulmonary function in patients with asthma or COPD (Poole & Black, 2000).

The majority of studies of NAC in lung disease used the oral form. Aerosolized NAC can, theoretically, disrupt the mucin layer, interfering with normal mucus clearance and airway protection (Rubin, 2007). Aerosolized NAC can irritate the airways and produce bronchoconstriction in patients with hyperactive airways. Aerosolized and oral forms of NAC appear to be inactivated in the airway or do not get into the mucus. Double-blind, placebo-controlled, randomized studies of mucolytics are few, but based on current data and results of published meta-analyses, the American Thoracic Society does not recommend mucolytics in the management of asthma or COPD (1995); therefore, the use of NAC is not recommended in patients with ALS who need assistance with secretion mobilization until more research is conducted.

Expectorants

Expectorants increase the volume of airway secretions. Expectorants are intended to improve movement of mucus from the larger airways to the oropharynx, where it can be swallowed or ejected. Although not a precise term, expectorant generally refers to a medication or other substance that increases airway water, volume of secretions, surfactants (that deter secretions from adhering to airway walls), and overall hydration. The most common expectorants are simple hydration (ingestion of liquids or inhaled bland aerosols) and glyceryl guaiacolate (guaifenesin) (Rubin, 2007).

Hydration is often recommended when secretions appear thick and tenacious and difficult to mobilize, especially if the patient is dehydrated and fluid intake is suboptimal. It is thought that dry, tenacious secretions adhere to airway walls, making them harder to remove by coughing; however, systemic hydration also does not appear to impact inspissated secretions, and there is not a good method of rehydrating the surface of dry secretions. In addition, these methods do not improve ciliary or mucosal efficiency in removing secretions.

Guaifenesin, marketed as Robatussin and Mucinex, is an expectorant that has been widely prescribed to alleviate cough since the 1950s. In fact, the Robins company has produced and sold cough preparations based on glyceryl ether of guaiacol since 1905. The benefits of guaifenesin are thought to derive from its ability to increase sputum volume and decrease sputum viscosity. Guaifenesin stimulates the cholinergic pathway and increases mucus secretion from the submucosal glands. It may inhibit cough reflex sensitivity in patients with upper respiratory infection and transient hypersensitivity and upper airway irritability (Dicpingaitis & Gayle, 2003).

That guaifenesin is safe when taken orally is not in dispute; however, clinical data to support its efficacy in sputum removal are conflicting. In 1976, the Food and Drug Administration set out to test the myriad of over-the-counter drugs for efficacy. At that time, guaifenesin was not shown to be effective in clearing airway secretions (Sharfstein et al., 1976). In 1989, a placebo-controlled clinical evaluation of guaimesal was undertaken by Jager (1989) and showed no significant difference between medication and placebo. Recently, guaifenesin has increased in popularity as an over-the-counter expectorant, now marketed as Mucinex, and has received Food and Drug Administration approval for an extended release compound with and without pseudoephedrine.

Again, because studies remain inconclusive clinicians should proceed with caution.

Expectorants are most frequently recommended when patients are troubled by a nonproductive cough. By increasing the volume of airway secretions, the effectiveness of the cough appears to be improved as the patient now has "something to show for it." RCPs are encouraged to explore the etiology of a cough, to determine whether increased sputum production is due to infection, and if retained secretions are due to hypoventilation and impaired cough.

Medications purported to increase secretion volume and antitussive agents (such as dextromethorphan) should not be prescribed together (Rubin, 2007). ALS patients with impaired coughing caused by expiratory and bulbar muscle weakness should use expectorants with caution.

Mucokinetic Agents

Mucokinetic agents increase the kinesis (movement) of mucus enhancing the mucociliary escalator and assisting the transportation of mucus from the airway (Rogers, 2007). Bronchodilator medications such as B-agonists and methylxanthines increase ciliary beat frequency, but have not been shown to significantly improve mucociliary clearance (Rubin, 2007). Bronchodilators may increase airway secretions and are not recommended for patients with weakened respiratory muscles and impaired cough. If a patient with ALS has a history of reactive airway disease that shows reversibility on pulmonary function after bronchodilator administration, this concomitant disease should be closely followed and managed following the Global Initiative for Chronic Obstructive Lung Disease guidelines (www.goldcopd.org) or the current National Institutes of Health guidelines for asthma management (http://www.nhlbi.nih.gov/guidelines/asthgdln).

LOWER RESPIRATORY TRACT INFECTIONS

Challenges to Identifying Pathogens

People with ALS are strongly encouraged to be immunized for annual flu strains and pneumococcal pneumonia. To insure adherence to this recommendation, multidisciplinary ALS clinics may choose to vaccinate patients during routine visits. Risk of hospitalization caused by lower respiratory infection becomes greater as the disease progresses. Nevertheless, patients may present in the clinic with cough and sputum production, with or without fever. Because of the emergence of antibiotic-resistant bacteria, physicians may be reluctant to prescribe antibiotics unless a respiratory tract pathogen is identified. It has long been the role of RCPs to obtain and document the color, consistency, and quantity of expectorated sputum from the lower respiratory tract when pneumonia is suspected. The quality of the sample can be discussed with the physician and a decision made to order gram stain and culture or treat empirically.

It has been common wisdom in respiratory therapy circles to assume that cream, white, or clear colored sputum is free of bacteria, whereas yellow, green, or yellow-green color is the result of infection. Sputum samples do not always produce reliable data because of contamination with oral flora, because they are not guaranteed to be from the lower respiratory tract, or because they may not contain the pathogen responsible for the infection. Sputum color in the yellow to green range (purulent) is typically the result of inflammatory cell-derived DNA, sloughed mucosal epithelial cells (cell debris), and degenerating neutrophils. Purulent secretions can be the result of viral or bacterial infection. Even if sputum samples are submitted for microbiologic analysis, false-positive and false-negative results are high (Tobin, 1987). In a recent study of 144 acceptable lower-respiratory tract sputum specimens, samples were rated by color and compared with Gram stain and culture results (Johnson et al., 2007). Study results showed a clear relationship between purulent sputum color and the acceptability of Gram-stain quality and microbiological findings. More research needs to be done in this area, but this study reinforces the trend toward identification of specific organisms in sputum before prescribing antibiotics known to treat them and the usefulness of color as an initial screening tool before laboratory testing.

SUMMARY

Respiratory therapy students spend a minimum of 18 months focused on the lower airway in all of its complexity. The lungs, their normal function and pathology, remain an exciting area of research and practice long after graduation. The more that is learned about the lung's intricacies, the more apparent are the gaps in our knowledge. RCPs who join the staff of a multidisciplinary ALS clinic or who work with people diagnosed with ALS in the home or acute-care setting draw on basic pulmonary assessment skills. Familiarity with respiratory pharmacology and techniques for managing respiratory insufficiency and infection is essential. Because controlled studies in managing cough, secretion retention, and respiratory insufficiency in ALS are lacking or few, RCPs must draw from classic pulmonary diseases to guide patient care and recommendations to physicians. Translating knowledge of chronic and acute lung diseases to neuromuscular disease often calls for educated guesswork based on experience and opinion. Creativity and open-minded skepticism are essential. This is most apparent in discussing expectorants, mucolytics, and mucokinetics in ALS.

REFERENCES

American Thoracic Society. Standards for the diagnosis and care of patients with chronic obstructive pulmonary disease. *Am J Respir Crit Care Med* 1995;152 (Suppl 1):S1–S21.

Anneser J, Borasio GD. Symptom control in amyotrophic lateral sclerosis/motor neuron disease. In Shaw P, Strong M (eds.). *Motor Neuron Disorders.* Philadelphia: Butterworth and Heinemann; 2003, pp. 485–496.

Boitano L. Management of airway clearance in neuromuscular disease. *Respiratory Care* 2006;51:913–922.

Carden D, Mathay M, George R. Functional anatomy of the respiratory system. In George R, Light R, Matthay M, Matthay R (eds.). *Chest Medicine: Essentials of Pulmonary and Critical Care.* Philadelphia: Lippincott Williams & Wilkins; 2005, pp. 3–23.

Corren J. The link between allergic rhinitis and asthma, otitis media, sinusitis and nasal polyps. *Immnunol Allergy Clin North Am* 2000;20:205.

Dantzker DR. Lung anatomy and development. In Dantzker D, MacIntyre N, Bakow E (eds.). *Comprehensive Respiratory Care.* Philadelphia: W.B. Saunders; 1995, pp. 1–17.

Decramer M, Rutten-van Molken M, Dekhuijzen PN, et al. Effects of N-acetylcysteine on outcomes in chronic obstructive pulmonary disease: a randomized placebo-controlled trial. *Lancet* 2005;365:1552–1560.

Dicpingaitis PV, Gayle YE. Effects of guaifenesin on cough reflex sensitivity. *Chest* 2003;124:2178–2181.

Donahue J. Safety and efficacy of B agonists. *Respiratory Care* 2008;53: 618–624.

Expert Panel Report 3: Guidelines for the Diagnosis and Management of Asthma. Bethesda, MD: National Institutes of Health, National Asthma Education and Prevention Program; 2007. NIH Publication No. 08-4051. Available from http://www.nhlbi.nih.gov/guidelines/asthgdln.pdf.

Irwin RS, Madison JM. The diagnosis and treatment of cough. *N Engl J Med* 2000;343:1715–1721.

Irwin RS, Baumann MH, Bolser DC, et al. American College of Chest Physicians (ACCP). Diagnosis and management of cough: ACCP evidence-based clinical practice guidelines. *Chest* 2006;129(1 Suppl):1S–23S.

Jager EG. Double-blind, placebo-controlled clinical evaluation of guaimesal in outpatients. *Clin Ther* 1989;11:107–111.

Johnson AL, Hampson DF, Hampson NB. Sputum color: implications for clinical practice. *Respiratory Care* 2007;53:450–454.

King CS, Moores LK. Clinical asthma syndromes and important asthma mimics. *Respiratory Care* 2008;53:568–582.

King M, Rubin BK. Rheology: relationship with transport. In Takishima T (ed.). *Airway Secretion: Physiological Bases for the Control of Hypersecretion.* New York: Marcel Dekker; 1994, pp. 283–314.

Lee J. Allergic rhinitis. *AARC Times* 2008;32:28–29.

Manterola C, Munoz S, Grande L, Bustos L. Initial validation of a questionnaire for detecting gastroesophageal reflux disease in the epidemiological setting. *J Clin Epidemiol* 2002;55:1042–1045.

Naclerio R, Solomon W. Rhinitis and inhalant allergens. *JAMA* 1997;278: 1842–1848.

Poole PJ, Black PN. Mucolytic agents for chronic bronchitis or chronic obstructive pulmonary disease. *Cochrane Database Syst Rev* 2000;(2):CD001287.

Redington AE, Morice AH (eds.). *Acute and Chronic Cough.* Boca Raton, FL: Taylor & Francis; 2005.

Rogers DF. Physiology of airway secretion and pathophysiology of hypersecretion. *Respiratory Care* 2007;52:1134–1149.

Rubin BK. Mucolytics, expectorants, and mucokinetic medications. *Respiratory Care* 2007;52:859–865.

Rubin BK, Hess DR. Forward to airway clearance: physiology, pharmacology, techniques, and practice. *Respiratory Care* 2007;52:1132–1133.

Sharfstein JM, North M, Serwint JR. Over the counter but no longer under the radar: pediatric cough and cold medications. *N Engl J Med* 1976;357:232–234.

Sheffner AL, Medler EM, Jacobs LW, Sarett HP. The in vitro reduction in viscosity of human tracheobronchial secretions by acetylcysteine. *Am Rev Respir Dis* 1964;90:721–729.

Sobande PO, Kercsmar CM. Inhaled corticosteroids in asthma management. *Respiratory Care* 2008;53:625–634.

Tobin MJ. Diagnosis of pneumonia: techniques and problems. *Clin Chest Med* 1987;8:513–527.

van der Schans CP. Bronchial transport. *Respiratory Care* 2007;52:1150–1158.

QUESTIONS FOR RESEARCH

1. Is guaifenesin effective for patients with nonproductive cough caused by an upper respiratory tract infection or upper-airway cough syndrome?

2. In determining the effectiveness of a mucolytic or other pharmacologic intervention for secretion mobilization, how will the rate of mucus clearance be quantified?

3. How can a dry cough in response to airway irritation be distinguished from a dry cough in response to lower-airway infection?

4. Are mechanical methods of mucolysis (internal or external vibration) more effective than drugs for thinning mucus?

CHAPTER 5

Clinical Respiratory Assessment of ALS

CHAPTER OUTLINE

CASE HISTORY

The medical director of the intensive care unit requested a neurologic consultation for Mrs. Alvarez, a 59-year-old woman who had exhibited altered mental status and developed respiratory failure after outpatient colonoscopy for iron-deficiency anemia. The respiratory care practitioners (RCPs) reported difficulty weaning her from mechanical ventilation, although she appeared medically stable and no underlying pulmonary or cardiac pathology could be determined.

History of Present Illness

Mrs. Alvarez underwent a colonoscopy on October 12th, was transferred to the emergency department after becoming obtunded, and was admitted to the intensive care unit (ICU) in the early hours of October 13th after developing hypercarbic respiratory failure. Her arterial blood gases drawn in the emergency department showed a pH of 7.075 and PCO_2 of 141. Her blood pressure was 197/97, and her heart rate was 104. Her respiratory rate was 20, and her oxygen saturation was 100% on 4 L/m of oxygen. Notes indicated that she had received Versed and fentanyl, drugs that can lead to respiratory suppression. Narcan and flumazenil were administered in an attempt to reverse these medications but were unsuccessful. She had been intubated, placed on mechanical ventilation, and transferred to the ICU.

During her 19 days in ICU, multiple attempts at extubation had been followed by respiratory distress and reintubation. Physician progress notes suggested that initially her difficulty weaning was attributed to a combination of medications and to a history of chronic obstructive pulmonary disease. After 10 days of failed attempts to extubate, a tracheostomy was performed. A neurologic consultation was requested.

When assessed in the ICU by the neurologist, Mrs. Alvarez was not on any medications that would suppress respirations. She had been successfully treated for a mild bronchial infection and an *Escherichia coli* urinary tract infection. A bronchoscopy showed no airway abnormalities. Mucus plugging in the left main stem bronchus had been resolved, and the lung successfully re-expanded. Chest radiography was notable only for an elevated left hemidiaphragm. Her pulmonary status appeared to be essentially normal.

Past Medical History

A gastric carcinoma had been resected 6 months before. Mrs. Alvarez had lost approximately 50 pounds in the 6 months after surgery because of difficulties with her jejunostomy tube and inadequate enteral feedings. She stated that she had had difficulty swallowing since her surgery but attributed it to intubation during surgery and not to any discrete condition. She denied difficulty walking or using her arms. Since being bedridden in the ICU she reported generalized weakness in arms and legs. After further questioning, she admitted to mild right-hand weakness before the colonoscopy. She denied difficulty breathing before acute respiratory failure after colonoscopy. She denied difficulty with sensation or with her bowel or bladder. She reported no pain.

Mrs. Alvarez had a history of diabetes and hypertension, both well controlled. Her medications included Advair, Combivent, and albuterol for treatment of mild chronic obstructive pulmonary disease (COPD).

Social History
Mrs. Alvarez was widowed and lived alone. She had three adult children who lived nearby and with whom she had frequent contact and good rapport.

Neurologic Examination
Three possible causes of respiratory failure and an inability to wean from mechanical ventilation were suspected: myasthenia gravis or a demyelinating neuropathy, amyotrophic lateral sclerosis, and neural carcinomatosis, the widespread dissemination of carcinoma. Motor studies and an electromyography (EMG) were performed. The neurologist noted generalized atrophy. The EMG showed a pattern of denervation throughout the upper extremities and fasciculations in areas of the lower extremities. These finding were consistent with amyotrophic lateral sclerosis (ALS). Results of a lumbar puncture ruled out disseminated malignancy of the cancer.

Discharge Summary
Mrs. Alvarez was diagnosed with amyotrophic lateral sclerosis with respiratory failure. She was transferred to a transitional care unit where the family was trained in tracheostomy care and ventilator management. She was discharged home with long-term mechanical ventilation. Mrs. Alvarez moved in with a daughter who shared caregiving responsibilities with her siblings. Mild chronic anemia, hypertension, mild COPD, and

diabetes were stabilized before discharge. Jejunostomy was functioning well, and her nutritional status had greatly improved. Mrs. Alvarez had elected to remain a "full code" and wanted to be resuscitated in the event of acute cardiac or respiratory failure. She was referred to a multidisciplinary ALS clinic. Neurologists continued to follow her progress, and allied health professionals evaluated her for motorized wheelchair with portable ventilator attachments. Home safety evaluations were made, and recommendations for improving mobility and reducing muscle contractures were offered. Mrs. Alvarez, a positive person by nature, continued to enjoy the company of her children, grandchildren, friends, and neighbors.

INTRODUCTION

Respiratory assessment of the neuromuscular patient includes ventilation, airway protection, and airway clearance. The initial visit to the neuromuscular clinic and all subsequent visits should include a detailed respiratory assessment. This assessment includes objective measures (pulmonary function, heart rate, respiratory rate, and body weight), observed symptoms (chest movement, palpation, and speech), and subjective measures of respiratory function (dyspnea, fatigue, and sleep quality). Determining patient's understanding and perceptions of their disease and ramifications of respiratory compromise is useful. Perceptions of spouses, partners, family members, and caregivers are useful because patients may underreport or minimize their symptoms. Consistency in assessment will also allow clinicians to compare changes in patient symptoms over time. A sample respiratory assessment form can be found in Appendix 5-1 at the end of this chapter.

In ALS, the primary cause of ventilatory failure and respiratory symptoms is inspiratory muscle weakness (Heffernan et al., 2006); however, the best test for determining early respiratory insufficiency has not been established (Miller et al., 1999). No single test of muscle strength has been shown to predict hypoventilation and carbon dioxide retention reliably (Lyall et al., 2001). Forced vital capacity and diurnal $SpO2$ measures may remain normal even in the face of nocturnal hypoventilation. At this time, a combination of clinical respiratory assessment and objective measures of lung function are the most effective methods of monitoring ALS progression. Clinicians are advised to check for signs and symptoms of early respiratory insufficiency routinely and perform serial measurements of pulmonary function (Heffernan et al., 2006).

ALS FUNCTIONAL RATING SCORE

Patients managed in multidisciplinary neuromuscular centers receive a score on each visit reflecting their overall stability or decline in function. The ALS functional rating score (ALSFRS-R) contains 12 areas of assessment, three of which are specific to respiratory function (Appendix 5-2). Patients are asked to rate their degree of orthopnea, dyspnea, and use of noninvasive positive pressure ventilation (NPPV) and are scored from 0 (severe) to 4 (absent). As disease progresses, scores fall (Cedarbaum et al., 1999). Of course, quantifying symptoms using ALSFRS-R do not replace a detailed pulmonary assessment but do assist in research and gaining an overall picture of patient symptoms, their correlation to test data, and disease course.

RESPIRATORY INSUFFICIENCY: SIGNS, SYMPTOMS, AND SIGNIFICANCE

Clinician observation of respiratory function and patient-reported symptoms will fall into three main categories: those that are measured (respiratory rate, heart rate, and weight), those that are observed (muscle use, speech rate, and pattern of speech), and patient perceptions (shortness of breath, fatigue, and sleep quality). Signs and symptoms of respiratory insufficiency can be subtle, and thus, clinicians should ask detailed questions that are suggestive of early respiratory muscle weakness (Lechtzin et al., 2002). The following are signs and symptoms of respiratory insufficiency that should prompt additional evaluation and testing. They are covered in greater detail later in this chapter along with their significance in ALS.

Symptoms of Respiratory Insufficiency

- Dyspnea on exertion
- Dyspnea while supine
- Dyspnea at rest
- Excessive fatigue
- Excessive daytime sleepiness
- Frequent nocturnal awakenings
- Morning headaches
- Nightmares
- Anxiety
- Cognitive impairment

Adapted from Heffernan et al. (2006).

Signs of Respiratory Insufficiency

- Reduced chest expansion
- Accessory muscle use at rest
- Inability to speak in full sentences
- Inability to project one's voice
- Tachypnea
- Weak cough
- Weak sniff
- Paradoxical inward movement of the abdomen on inspiration

Adapted from Heffernan et al. (2006)

Measures of Cardiopulmonary Dysfunction

Heart Rate and Respiratory Rate

Tachypnea and tachycardia at rest can be signs of respiratory insufficiency. In diaphragmatic muscle fatigue, as measured by EMG, the ratio of high-frequency electrical activity to low-frequency electrical activity decreases (Cohen et al., 1982). This correlates clinically with an increased respiratory rate and is observed as rapid, shallow breathing. Laboratory measures show decreased $PaCO_2$ and $ETCO_2$ levels in the early stages of respiratory muscle weakness. In patients with neuromuscular disease, the ratio of respiratory rate to tidal volume (f/V_T) is a useful measure of respiratory muscle fatigue. Patients with neuromuscular disease use a greater percentage of ventilatory reserve than normal patients. Without intervention to reduce the work of breathing and rest ventilatory muscles, respiratory muscle fatigue will lead to respiratory failure as $PaCO_2$ levels rise.

The heart and lungs work in tandem to meet the body's metabolic needs—the muscles' need for oxygen. In healthy individuals, increased tissue oxygenation is achieved through increased minute ventilation and increased cardiac output during exercise. A restrictive lung pattern on pulmonary function tests with a decreased minute ventilatory volume is seen in patients with ALS. Because of a lack of ventilatory reserves, increased lung volume in response to exercise is not possible. In order to maintain the ventilation-to-perfusion ratio the respiratory rate will increase. The patient experiences the lack of pulmonary reserves as exertional dyspnea. In addition, the body's attempt to maintain adequate oxygenation in response to increased metabolic needs and hypoxemia will result in increased heart rate and, in some cases, cardiac dysrhythmias.

If ALS is progressing slowly, patients may not experience acute dyspnea or be aware of the presence of compensatory mechanisms. Decreased exercise tolerance may be attributed to diagnoses other than early neuro-muscular disease, such as general muscle deconditioning or depression. Limited mobility and decreased physical activity caused by wheelchair dependence or an inability to climb stairs or walk up inclines can mask lung impairment. Over time, to conserve energy and spare further respira-tory muscle fatigue, the body may accept an altered baseline of PaO_2 and $PaCO_2$. Patients who have acclimated to low resting tidal volumes may have a difficult time adjusting to nocturnal use of NPPV, as morning discontinuance of assisted ventilation will bring about a period of dyspnea as the body readjusts to low volumes once again. Difficult adjustment to noninvasive assisted ventilation in later stages of ALS is one reason an increasing number of RCPs, physicians, nurses, and other health care professionals advocate for early treatment with NPPV before symptoms become severe.

Hemoglobin and hematocrit levels should be checked if vital capacity measures do not fully explain elevation of heart and respiratory rate. As respiratory muscles weaken, increased work of breathing will increase oxygen demand. If hemoglobin is decreased or inadequate for the amount of oxygen needed, the imbalance will result in fatigue, weakness, and dyspnea.

Body Weight and Dehydration

Weight should be measured on initial and all subsequent clinic visits. Weight loss in ALS is often caused by a loss of muscle mass. Diaphragmatic muscle weakness, accessory muscle use, and compensatory tachypnea create a situation in which energy (caloric) expenditure exceeds supply. A hypermetabolic state can contribute to weight loss and insidious, progressive malnutrition. Protein deficiency is usually the result of caloric deficiency. Protein catabolism and a loss of muscle mass results in weakness and lethargy. Serum albumin is reduced in prolonged protein deficiency.

Much of the research on nutrition and respiratory muscles has been conducted in COPD (Donahoe et al., 1989; Lewis & Belman, 1988). In a study comparing malnourished patients with COPD, well-nourished patients with COPD, and normal controls, resting energy requirements and oxygen cost of breathing were significantly elevated in the malnourished group (Donahoe et al.). Even when caloric intake is not reduced weight loss can be attributed to decreased efficiency of respiratory muscles and increased work of breathing (Lewis & Belman). Lewis and Belman observed atrophy of type 2 muscle fibers with malnutrition. As type 2 fibers are responsible for most of the force exerted by the muscle, one may make the link between malnutrition and muscle weakness (Dantzker, 1995).

Arora and Rochester (1982) studied the negative affect of weight loss on pulmonary function. They found marked reductions in PI_{max}, vital capacity, and maximal voluntary ventilation in patients whose ideal body weight was 71% of normal. Results of nutritional intervention on pulmonary function studies, morbidity, and mortality in non-ALS patients are not conclusive (Dantzker, 1995). In ALS, there is no conclusion regarding the benefit of enteral nutrition on mortality or quality of life (Miller et al., 1999).

Inadequate fluid intake may result when patients fear choking and aspirating thin liquids because of bulbar muscle weakness. Decreased skin turgor is the principal clinical sign, but elevated hematocrit, plasma creatinine, and blood urea nitrogen levels can also signal inadequate fluid intake. If difficulty chewing and swallowing is hindering adequate food and fluid intake, speech language pathologists can suggest a range of solutions from head and neck positioning to thickening agents for liquids. Registered dietitians assess patients' food preferences and caloric needs and recommend diets and supplements rich in protein, fats, and carbohydrates.

Observed Symptoms

Chest Movement

Normal Breathing

Observation of chest expansion and muscle use should be assessed in ALS. In early or moderate respiratory insufficiency, respiratory examination is likely to be normal. Pattern and effort of breathing, thoracic configuration, and lung expansion are assessed visually. Assessment is best with patient sitting upright in a well-lighted room. In normal diaphragmatic breathing, the abdomen moves out slightly on inhalation and back to resting on exhalation. Rate and rhythm are consistent at 12 to 20 breaths per minute.

Accessory Muscle Use

Progressive diaphragm weakness can lead to activation and improved mechanical efficiency of accessory muscles, even at rest. As the diaphragm and intercostals (primary muscles of ventilation) lose innervation, accessory muscles can assist ventilation by raising the anterior chest to increase lung volume.

The inspiratory neck muscles—the scalenes—elevate the first and second ribs and pull the chest upward on inhalation. Activation of inspiratory neck muscles during resting inspiration is called the respiratory pulse. Along with abdominal paradox (inward movement of the abdomen on inhalation), observation of a respiratory pulse is a sign of severe diaphragm muscle weakness (Similowski et al., 2000).

The sternomastoid muscles are attached to the clavicle and the sternum. These upper rib cage muscles assist in ventilation by elevating the first rib and the sternum, moving the chest forward. The pectoralis major is attached to the middle of the clavicle, the sternum, and the upper six costal cartilages. By stabilizing the arms and shoulders, patients can use the pectoralis major muscle to increase the diameter of the chest by lifting the sternum and ribs. Some patients can maintain an FVC above 50% by using accessory muscles to assist the diaphragm; therefore, additional measures of pulmonary function (maximum inspiratory pressure, sniff negative inspiratory pressure) more specific to the diaphragm should be routinely obtained.

Compensatory Mechanisms

Paradoxical movement of the diaphragm refers to inward movement on inspiration. This occurs when negative thoracic pressure generated by contraction of accessory muscles pulls a flaccid diaphragm upward. When the diaphragm is partially weakened, clinicians may observe alternating use of the diaphragm and accessory muscles, referred to as respiratory alternans.

In severe diaphragmatic weakness, the abdominal muscles can also contribute to inspiration. When contracted at end exhalation, increased intra-abdominal pressure pushes the diaphragm upward, the lower rib cage inflates, the chest wall stores energy, and elastic recoil assists in the next inspiration. Some patients ventilate adequately as long as abdominal and accessory muscles remain functional and, having compensated over time, may not complain of debilitating dyspnea. Weakening of abdominal muscles and muscles of the upper chest in this subgroup of ALS patients will lead to respiratory failure and the eventual need for continuous non-invasive or invasive ventilation.

Palpation

Palpation may be used to assess lung movement. If diaphragmatic, accessory, and abdominal muscle movement are difficult to observe, clinicians may place hands over muscle groups to judge expansion. Placing hands over the posterior lower rib cage with thumbs at midline allows one to visualize the degree of thoracic expansion and whether movement of the diaphragm is equal bilaterally. Unilateral movement may be due to unequal innervation of the right and left diaphragm, localized atelectasis, or infiltrates. Independent movement of upper and lower rib cage and subtle movement of the abdomen may be better detected through touch than visual inspection.

Speech Rate and Pattern

Word generation and voice projection are observable signs of pulmonary muscle weakness. As the diaphragm weakens, expiratory flow through the vocal cords is reduced. This results in reduced volume, and thus, a patient may be difficult to hear. The work of breathing may increase as patients try to project their voice. Patients may speak in short phrases because of decreased tidal volume. Patients may adapt by inhaling to their maximum capacity and speaking only on exhalation. The number of words a patient can generate in 1 minute is documented by speech language pathologists on each clinic visit and is another indicator of respiratory muscle strength as well as upper airway function. Assessment techniques used by speech language pathologists are detailed in Chapter 3. Volume expansion techniques and noninvasive mechanical ventilation with angled mouthpiece to assist in voice projection are discussed in Chapter 7.

Patient Reported Symptoms

Overview

Shortness of breath, fatigue, and sleep quality are subjective symptoms that clinicians use to infer pulmonary muscle function. Combined with objective and clinical measures, patient reported symptoms complete the picture. Patients' perceptions of their symptoms and successful adaptations to diminished pulmonary function affect quality of life. The clinician's role is to take the time to elicit symptoms, let patients share how they feel in their own words, and listen objectively and without preconceived conceptions. After patients know that they have been heard and understood, they will be in a better position to hear clinician recommendations for symptom relief and disease management. Assisted ventilation is often discussed during the initial respiratory assessment. Some patients are ready for this discussion early in the disease course. Others choose to defer discussion of respiratory support while they absorb the ramifications of their diagnosis. Clinicians will take their clue from the patients about appropriate timing of these discussions; however, early education about respiratory symptom management has been shown to be successful in avoiding emergency intubation and tracheostomy in patients with ALS (McKim, 2007).

**Clinician Guide to Patient Assessment and
Treatment Management**

L *Listen* with sympathy and understanding to the patient's perceptions
E *Explain* your perception of the problem
A *Acknowledge* and discuss the differences and similarities in perceptions
R *Recommend* treatment
N *Negotiate* agreement

Berlin & Fowkes (1983).

Dyspnea

Dyspnea, the perception of breathlessness, is by definition subjective. It is how patients experience respiratory muscle fatigue. The presence of dyspnea is a primary factor affecting quality of life and a major source of discomfort in ALS. In the "History of Dyspnea," a distinction is made between the terms dyspnea and breathlessness (Killian, 2005). Dyspnea is the sensation of increased effort that occurs during the act of breathing. Breathlessness describes discomfort that accompanies the urge to breathe. Patients may describe the experience as "breathing through a straw" or as if they are "holding their breath." Dyspnea is part perception of the sensation of breathlessness and part reaction to the sensation (Stulbarg & Carrieri-Kohlman, 1992).

Dyspnea is an inspiratory phenomenon. It stems from a multitude of factors, but in patients with neuromuscular disease, it is often the result of decreased total lung volume, increased residual volume, a loss of muscle mass strength, inadequate caloric intake, and choking due to loss of upper airway innervation. In response to hypoxemia or hypercapnia, the central nervous system signals the diaphragm and intercostals to contract in order to generate greater respiratory rate and lung volumes (minute ventilation). In ALS, signals from the central nervous system to activate respiratory muscles are not successfully transmitted. It is hypothesized that weak respiratory muscles create a discrepancy between effort to breathe and inadequate response; therefore, the greater the signal, the greater is the dyspnea experienced (Carrieri et al., 1984).

In acute respiratory insufficiency (increased $PaCO_2$ and decreased pH), the inability of the respiratory muscles to respond to carotid body stimulation (drive to breathe) creates the sensation of dyspnea. Very small changes in $PaCO_2$ can induce a large degree of breathlessness; however, patients who have compensated respiratory acidosis (chronically elevated $PaCO_2$ levels, increased base excess, and normalized pH), carotid body stimulation may be blunted and sensation of breathless reduced (Bloch-Salisbury et al., 1996).

Reported dyspnea in patients newly diagnosed with ALS should prompt pulmonary function tests. Measurement of vital capacity and maximum inspiratory pressure is essential. Neurologists may test EMG response to phrenic nerve stimulation (Similowski et al., 2000).

Dyspnea with exertion is one of the early symptoms of ALS. As the disease progresses, patients experience dyspnea at rest. This can prompt great emotional distress in patients, as there is less that they can do to alleviate the symptom. Patients often reduce physical activity to avoid dyspnea. Once unable to walk or wheelchair dependent, patients may not experience dyspnea to a great degree; however, a lack of reported dyspnea in this population can mask continued decline in lung function.

ALSFRS-R scores dyspnea based on situations during which it occurs: at rest, while talking, or while eating, dressing, or bathing. Functional rating scores are useful in assessing patient response to disease progression. Scales that determine breathing discomfort during activities of daily living are one measure of quality of life, which is of great importance to ALS patients, their families, clinicians who work with them, and increasingly in research. Visual analogue scales have not been used consistently in multidisciplinary centers (e.g., 10-point scale with 0 = "no breathing difficulty" to 10 = "extreme breathing difficulty") A new study by Just et al. (2007) advocates using such an instrument, the Borg dyspnea score, to predict inspiratory muscle weakness in ALS. Using a modified Borg score of 0 = "no breathing difficulty" and 5 = "extreme breathing difficulty," they found that a score of 3 was significantly related to SNIP pressure ≤ -40 cm H_2O and a score ≥ 3 correlated significantly with lower inspiratory muscle strength and slightly higher $PaCO_2$.

Dyspnea has been studied extensively in patients with obstructive lung disease, and most dyspnea-rating scales are developed with this population in mind. Clearly, dyspnea scales that assess breathlessness created by exertion, such as walking or stair climbing, are not useful in a patient population with limited mobility. Lechtzin et al. (2007) evaluated measures of dyspnea in patients with ALS. They found the baseline dyspnea index and transitional dyspnea index useful in ALS as these scales do not inquire about specific physical tasks (Appendix 5-3). They also found that the transitional dyspnea index significantly correlated with changes in FVC in patients with mild to moderate respiratory impairment.

More research needs to be undertaken to correlate measures of pulmonary function with subjective symptoms of respiratory insufficiency. Lechtzin et al. (2007) have contributed to this research and recommend the baseline dyspnea index/transitional dyspnea index (Mahler et al., 1984) for sensitivity to changes in dyspnea over time, reproducibility, ease of administration, and as an improvement on the ALSFRS-R respiratory subscale in measuring breathlessness.

Orthopnea

Orthopnea is the inability to comfortably lie down in a supine position. The degree of orthopnea is usually defined by the elevation of the head and upper body and is often expressed as "two-pillow" or "three-pillow" orthopnea. If using a hospital bed, one may refer to the head of the bed as being raised to the level of 30, 45, or 90 degrees, depending on patient need or comfort.

Orthopnea is a sign of diaphragmatic muscle weakness or reduced vital capacity. In the supine position, the abdominal contents move up, displacing a portion of the lungs. In addition, the positive effects of gravity on downward diaphragmatic excursion are lost. To compensate for nocturnal respiratory insufficiency, patients may sleep on their sides but will need to progress to an elevated position using pillows or foam wedge as the disease worsens. The presence of orthopnea in ALS is a marker of disease progression and is included in ALSFRS-R scoring.

Sleep-Disordered Breathing

Severe diaphragm dysfunction in ALS naturally leads to the problem of sleep-disordered breathing (Arnulf et al., 2000). The earliest signs of respiratory insufficiency in ALS may result from nocturnal hypoventilation (Ferguson et al., 1996). Patients may experience a host of symptoms that they do not identify as resulting from poor sleep quality: daytime fatigue, daytime sleepiness, frequent nighttime awakenings to urinate, morning headaches, poor concentration, short-term memory loss, irritability, depression, and anxiety. Sleep disruption in ALS can be caused by orthopnea, neuropathic pain, difficulty turning and changing position because of muscle weakness, periodic leg movement, muscle cramping, fasciculations, depression, anxiety, increased salivation and swallowing problems, or frequent urination (Ferguson et al.; Hetta & Jansson, 1997).

Diaphragmatic weakness is common in ALS, and patients compensate by using accessory muscles (scalenes and sternocleidomastoids) to assist inhalation. During rapid eye movement (REM) sleep, the restorative level of sleep, ventilation is accomplished almost solely through diaphragmatic movement. Accessory muscle assistance is inhibited. In an attempt to maintain adequate ventilation and oxygenation, ALS patients sacrifice REM sleep for lighter stages of sleep that allow for extradiaphragmatic muscle use. In a controlled prospective study of 21 patients with definite ALS, Arnulf et al. (2000) found that diaphragmatic dysfunction was associated with a dramatic reduction in REM sleep duration. A reduction in REM sleep results in altered sleep architecture and sleep fragmentation and is experienced as poor sleep quality.

Nocturnal oximetry studies may be useful in documenting SpO_2 changes that might be caused by nocturnal hypoventilation and account for daytime symptoms not attributed to other causes. Arnulf et al. found sleep disruption in ALS without significant hypoxemia and suggested that sustained awakenings were due to hypoventilation accompanied by rapid, shallow breathing. Clinicians should maintain a high degree of suspicion for sleep disordered breathing when patients present with these symptoms of sleep deprivation.

Epworth Sleepiness Scale

The Epworth Sleepiness Scale (ESS) is a validated self-administered questionnaire used to measure sleep deprivation and sleepiness in patients suspected to have obstructive sleep apnea. Although obstructive sleep apnea is generally not a problem in ALS patients, this scale can identify people who need assessment by a specialist in sleep disorders. Although short and simple to use, Weaver et al. (2004) caution against using the ESS as a surrogate for diagnosis of sleep disordered breathing. It can be used to screen for sleep deprivation and the need for overnight pulse oximetry study or polysomnography.

Subjects are asked to rate how likely they are to doze off in a variety of situations and rate that likelihood on a scale of 0 to 3, with 0 no chance of dozing and 3 a high chance of dozing. A score of 9 and above indicates sleep deprivation.

Dr. Murray Johns designed the ESS while working at the Epworth Sleep Center in Richmond, Victoria, Australia. It has been translated into many languages. Because the ESS is subjective, it may convey symptoms of fatigue rather than sleepiness. The ESS and rating scale follow:

Epworth Sleepiness Scale
Scoring

0 = no chance of dozing
1 = slight chance of dozing
2 = moderate chance of dozing
3 = high chance of dozing

Situation

- Sitting and reading
- Watching TV
- Sitting inactive in a public place (e.g., a theater or a meeting)
- As a passenger in a car for an hour without a break
- Lying down to rest in the afternoon when circumstances permit
- Sitting and talking to someone
- Sitting quietly after a lunch without alcohol
- In a car, while stopped for a few minutes in traffic

CO-MORBIDITIES

Pulmonary Disease

Patients may have underlying cardiopulmonary disease that predated the diagnosis of ALS. A thorough medical history will include the following:

- Pre-existing diagnoses of asthma, chronic bronchitis, or emphysema
- Past or current cigarette smoking
- Occupational exposure to pulmonary irritants
- Current respiratory medications

Consultation with the pulmonologist or primary care physician responsible for managing the patient's pulmonary disease will allow the RCP to share the ongoing results of clinic-based pulmonary function testing with them.

Diagnosed or suspected COPD will impact treatment choices and settings. For example, when initiating NPPV, inspiratory time, inspiratory-to-expiratory ratio, and rise time will need to be adjusted depending on the degree of airway compromise and air trapping.

Cardiovascular Disease

A patient history of cardiac or pulmonary hypertension, congestive heart failure, atrial or ventricular dysrhythmias, or a pacing device will impact assessment of vital signs and response to exertion. Having a baseline allows one to distinguish new symptoms from pre-existing ones. Lower-extremity weakness, limited mobility, and eventual confinement to wheelchair and bed put ALS patients at risk for deep vein thrombosis. Pulmonary embolism and resulting acute respiratory failure are underrecognized mortality risk factors for patients in the late stages of ALS.

SUMMARY

In the United States, ALS is classified as a restrictive pulmonary disease, as well as a disease of the motor neurons. Chronic alveolar hypoventilation and resulting structural changes in the pulmonary parenchyma result in increasing lung stiffness (Estenne et al., 1993). A decrease in the diameter of airways and alveoli results in increased airway resistance. For the patient with ALS, lung stiffness and decreased airflow manifest in increased work of breathing, dyspnea, sleep fragmentation, and fatigue. The role of RCPs is to assess the degree of lung function, elicit pulmonary symptoms, help patients manage symptoms, and maintain lung function for as long as possible.

REFERENCES

Arnulf I, Similowski T, Salachas F, et al. Sleep disorders and diaphragmatic function in patients with amyotrophic lateral sclerosis. *Am J Respir Crit Care Med* 2000; 161:849–856.

Arora NS, Rochester DF. Effect of body weight and muscularity on human diaphragm muscle mass, thickness, and area. *J Appl Physiol* 1982;52:64–70.

Berlin EA & Fowkes WC Jr. A teaching framework for cross-cultural health care: application in family practice. *West J Med* 1983;139:934–938.

Bloch-Salisbury E, Shea SA, Brown R, et al. Air hunger induced by acute increase in PCO_2 adapts to chronic elevation of PCO_2 in ventilated humans. *J Appl Physiol* 1996; 81(2):949–956.

Carrieri V, Jansen-Bjerklie S, Jacobs S. The sensation of dyspnea: a review. *Heart Lung J Crit Care* 1984;13:436–447.

Cedarbaum JM, Stambler N, Malta F, et al. The ALSFRS R: a revised ALS functional rating scale that incorporates assessments of respiratory function. *J Neurol Sci* 1999;169:13–21.

Cohen C, Zagelbaum G, Gross D, et al. Clinical manifestations of inspiratory muscle fatigue. *Am J Med* 1982;73:308–316.

Dantzker DR. Respiratory Muscles. In Dantzker DR, MacIntyre NR, Bakow ED (eds.). *Comprehensive Respiratory Care.* Philadelphia: W.B. Saunders; 1995, pp. 32–54.

Donahoe M, Rogers R, Wilson D, Pennock B. Oxygen consumption of the respiratory muscles in normal and malnourished patients with chronic obstructive pulmonary disease. *Am Rev Respir Dis* 1989;140:385–391.

Estenne M, Heilporn A, Delhez L, et al. Lung volume restriction in patients with chronic respiratory muscle weakness: the role of microatelectasis. *Thorax* 1993; 48:698–701.

Ferguson KA, Stong MA, Ahmad D, George CFP. Sleep-disordered breathing in amyotrophic lateral sclerosis. *Chest* 1996;110:664–669.

Heffernan C, Jenkinson C, Holmes T, et al. Management of respiration in MND/ALS patients: an evidence based review. *Amyotrophic Lateral Sclerosis* 2006; 7:5–15.

Hetta J, Jansson I. Sleep in patients with amyotrophic lateral sclerosis. *J Neurol* 1997;244(Suppl 1):S7–S9.

Just N, Bautin N, Daniel-Brunaud V, et al. The Borg dyspnea score: a relevant clinical marker of inspiratory muscle weakness in ALS. 2007. Unpublished manuscript.

Killian K. History of dyspnea. In Mahler DA, O'Donnell DE (eds.). *Dyspnea: Mechanisms, Measurement and Management.* Boca Raton, FL: Taylor and Francis; 2005, pp. 1–18.

Lechtzin N, Rothstein J, Clawson L, Diette GB, Wiener CM. Amyotrophic lateral sclerosis: evaluation and treatment of respiratory impairment. *Amyotrophic Lateral Sclerosis Other Motor Neuron Disord* 2002;3:5–13.

Lechtzin N, Lange D, Davey C, et al. Measures of dyspnea in patients with amyotrophic lateral sclerosis. *Muscle Nerve* 2007;35:98–102.

Lewis MI, Belman MJ. Nutrition and respiratory muscles. *Clin Chest Med* 1988;9:337–348.

Lyall RA, Donaldson N, Polkey MI, et al. Respiratory muscle strength and ventilatory failure in amyotrophic lateral sclerosis. *Brain* 2001;124:2000–2013.

Mahler DA, Weinberg DH, Wells CK, Feinstein AR. The measurement of dyspnea: contents, interobserver agreement, and physiologic correlates of two new clinical indexes. *Chest* 1984;85:751–758.

McKim DA. ALS Respiratory Care in Ottawa Canada. Presented at the ALS Association Will Rogers Institute Respiratory Symposium, Newport Beach, CA, January 2007.

Miller RG, Rosenberg JA, Gelinas DF, et al. Practice parameter: the care of the patient with amyotrophic lateral sclerosis (an evidence-based review): report of the Quality Standards Subcommittee of the American Academy of Neurology: ALS Practice Parameters Task Force. *Neurology* 1999;52:1311–1323.

Similowski T, Attali V, Bensimon G, et al. Diaphragmatic dysfunction and dyspnoea in amyotrophic lateral sclerosis. *Eur Respir J* 2000;15:332–337.

Stulbarg M, Carrieri-Kohlman V. Conceptual approach to the treatment of dyspnea: focus on the role of exercise. *Cardiopulmonary Physical Ther* 1992;3(1):9–11.

Weaver EM, Kapur V, Yueh B. Polysomnography vs self-reported measures in patients with sleep apnea (abstract). *Arch Otolaryngol Head Neck Surg* 2004;130: 453–458.

QUESTIONS FOR RESEARCH

1. What factors allow some ALS patients to use extradiaphragmatic muscles for inspiration (e.g., inspiratory neck muscles) when the diaphragm weakens while others do not?

2. What are the best methods for quantifying dyspnea in amyotrophic lateral sclerosis?

3. What are the best methods for treating the symptom of dyspnea in amyotrophic lateral sclerosis?

4. What personal variables are related to subjective symptoms of fatigue and dyspnea (e.g. age, gender, depression, anxiety, and social support)?

Respiratory Assessment

Name _____   Date _____

DOB _____   Diagnosis _____   ICD 9 Code _____

Pulmonary Test Results

Forced Vital Capacity (FVC) ____% Pred
Actual ____Liters Predicted ____Liters Upright

Forced Vital Capacity (FVC) ____% Pred
Actual ____Liters Predicted ____Liters Supine

Maximum Inspiratory Pressure (MIP) ____cm H_2O

SNIP ____cm H_2O

Peak Cough Flow ____LPM

SPO_2 ____% HR ____at rest SPO_2 ____% HR ____with ambulation

Distance ____ft   Recovery time ____minutes

Signs of Respiratory Insufficiency

Respiratory rate ____

Reduced chest expansion   ☐ Yes   ☐ No

Accessory muscle use at rest   ☐ Yes   ☐ No

Paradoxical abdominal movement   ☐ Yes   ☐ No

Poor appetite   ☐ Yes   ☐ No   Weight loss   ☐ Yes   ☐ No

Sleep Quality and Respiratory Symptomology

Number of hours of sleep per night _____ Number of awakenings _____
Perceived reason for awakenings

☐ nocturia   ☐ repositioning
☐ pain/discomfort   ☐ other

Need for daytime naps   ☐ Yes   ☐ No

Waking up in the morning feeling refreshed   ☐ Yes   ☐ No

Difficulty staying awake during the day   ☐ Yes   ☐ No

Waking up at night feeling like you were choking ☐ Yes   ☐ No

Waking up in the morning with a headache   ☐ Yes   ☐ No

Feeling short of breath when lying flat in bed   ☐ Yes   ☐ No

Difficulty concentrating or memory   ☐ Yes   ☐ No

Shortness of breath on exertion   ☐ Yes   ☐ No

Lack of energy or increased fatigue   ☐ Yes   ☐ No

Airway Clearance

Cough effectiveness _____ strong _____ fair _____ weak

Difficulty clearing secretions   ☐ Yes   ☐ No

Sialorrhea   ☐ Yes   ☐ No   Mucus   ☐ Yes   ☐ No

Respiratory History

Smoking History ☐ Yes ☐ No

Asthma ☐ Yes ☐ No; Bronchitis ☐ Yes ☐ No; Emphysema ☐ Yes ☐ No

Occupational exposure to pulmonary irritants ☐ Yes ☐ No

Respiratory Medications _____

Respiratory Assistive Devices

☐ Noninvasive Positive Pressure Ventilation (NPPV) Model _____
Settings _____

    Usage: Hours of use per night _____

        Hours used during the day _____

☐ Breath Stacking

    Usage: Number of times per day _____

☐ Cough Assist Device

    Usage: Number of times per day _____

☐ Suction unit

    Usage: Number of time per day _____

☐ Mechanical Ventilator

    Usage: Hours of usage _____

☐ Vest

    Usage: Number of times per day _____

☐ Other _____

Dyspnea 4 3 2 1 0   Orthopnea 4 3 2 1 0   Respiratory insufficiency 4 3 2 1 0

Comments/Suggestions:

RCP License #

ALSFRS-R

Type of Contact: Clinic Visit ☐   Phone Interview ☐

1. **SPEECH** ☐

   ☐ 4 normal speech processes
   ☐ 3 detectable speech disturbance
   ☐ 2 intelligible with repeating
   ☐ 1 speech combined with
      nonvocal communication
   ☐ 0 loss of useful speech

2. **SALIVATION** ☐

   ☐ 4 normal
   ☐ 3 slight but definite excess of
      saliva in mouth, may have
      nighttime drooling
   ☐ 2 moderately excessive saliva with
      some minimal drooling
   ☐ 1 marked excess of saliva with
      some drooling
   ☐ 0 marked drooling, requires
      constant tissue or handkerchief

3. **SWALLOWING** ☐

   ☐ 4 normal eating habits
   ☐ 3 early eating problems—
      occasional choking
   ☐ 2 dietary consistency changes
   ☐ 1 needs supplemental tube
      feeding
   ☐ 0 NPO (exclusively parenteral or
      enteral feeding)

4. **HANDWRITING** ☐

   ☐ 4 normal
   ☐ 3 slow or sloppy, all words legible
   ☐ 2 not all words are legible
   ☐ 1 able to grip pen but unable to
      write
   ☐ 0 unable to grip pen

5a. **CUTTING FOOD AND
   HANDLING UTENSILS** ☐

   (patients without gastrostomy)
   ☐ 4 normal
   ☐ 3 somewhat slow and clumsy but
      no help needed
   ☐ 2 can cut most foods, although
      clumsy and slow, some help
      needed
   ☐ 1 food must be cut by someone,
      but can still feed slowly
   ☐ 0 needs to be fed

5b. **CUTTING FOOD AND
   HANDLING UTENSILS** ☐

   (alternate scale for patients with
   gastrostomy)
   ☐ 4 normal
   ☐ 3 clumsy but able to perform all
      manipulations independently
   ☐ 2 some help needed with closures
      or fasteners
   ☐ 1 provides minimal assistance to
      caregiver
   ☐ 0 unable to perform any aspect of
      task

6. DRESSING AND HYGIENE ☐ ☐ 4 normal function ☐ 3 independent and complete self-care with effort or decreased efficiency ☐ 2 intermittent assistance or substitute methods ☐ 1 needs attendant for self care ☐ 0 total dependence	**10. DYSPNEA** ☐ ☐ 4 none ☐ 3 occurs when walking ☐ 2 occurs with one or more of the following: eating, bathing, dressing (ADLs) ☐ 1 occurs at rest, difficulty breathing when either sitting or lying ☐ 0 significant difficulty, considering using mechanical respiratory support
7. TURNING IN BED AND ADJUSTING BEDCLOTHES ☐ ☐ 4 normal ☐ 3 somewhat slow or clumsy, but no help needed ☐ 2 can turn alone or adjust sheets but with great difficulty ☐ 1 can initiate, but not turn or adjust sheets alone ☐ 0 helpless	**11. ORTHOPNEA** ☐ ☐ 4 none ☐ 3 some difficulty sleeping at night due to shortness of breath, does not routinely use more than two pillows ☐ 2 needs extra pillows in order to sleep (more than 2) ☐ 1 can only sleep sitting up ☐ 0 unable to sleep
8. WALKING ☐ ☐ 4 normal ☐ 3 early ambulation difficulties ☐ 2 walks with assistance ☐ 1 nonambulatory functional movement ☐ 0 no purposeful leg movement	**12. RESPIRATORY INSUFFICIENCY** ☐ ☐ 4 none ☐ 3 intermittent use of BiPAP ☐ 2 continuous use of BiPAP during the night ☐ 1 continuous use of BiPAP during the night and day ☐ 0 invasive mechanical ventilation by intubation or tracheostomy
9. CLIMBING STAIRS ☐ ☐ 4 normal ☐ 3 slow ☐ 2 mild unsteadiness or fatigue ☐ 1 needs assistance ☐ 0 cannot do	*TOTAL SCORE* _____

Place score for each section in the box (upper right-hand corner)

The Amyotrophic Lateral Sclerosis Functional Rating Scale. Assessment of activities of daily living in patients with amyotrophic lateral sclerosis. The ALS CNTF Treatment Study (ACTS) Phase I-II Study Group. *Arch Neurol* 1996;53:141–147.

Measures of Dyspnea

Measures of Dyspnea: Baseline Dyspnea Index (BDI) and Transitional Dyspnea Index (TDI). DA Mahler, 1984.

BASELINE DYSPNEA INDEX

Functional Impairment

Grade 4: No Impairment. Able to carry out usual activities and occupation without shortness of breath.

Grade 3: Slight impairment. Distinct impairment in at least one activity, but no activities completely abandoned. Reduction, in activity at work or in usual activities, that seems slight or not clearly caused by shortness of breath.

Grade 2: Moderate impairment. Patient has changed jobs and/or has abandoned at least one usual activity due to shortness of breath.

Grade 1: Severe impairment. Patient unable to work or has given up most or all usual activities due to shortness of breath.

Grade 0: Very severe impairment. Unable to work and has given up most or all usual activates due to shortness of breath.

W: Amount uncertain. Patient is impaired due to shortness of breath, but amount cannot be specified. Details are not sufficient to all impairment to be categorized.

X: Unknown. Information unavailable regarding impairment.

Y: Impaired for reasons other than shortness of breath—for example, musculoskeletal problems or chest pain.

Usual activities refer to requirements of daily living, maintenance or up keeping of residence, yard work, gardening, shopping, and so forth.

Magnitude of Task

Grade 4: Extraordinary. Becomes short of breath only with extraordinary activities such as carrying very heavy loads on the level, lighter loads uphill, or running. No shortness of breath with ordinary tasks.

Grade 3: Major. Becomes short of breath only with such major activities as walking up a steep hill, climbing more than three flights of stairs, or carrying a moderate load on the level.

Grade 2: Moderate. Becomes short of breath with moderate or average tasks such as walking up a gradual hill, climbing fewer than three flights of stairs, or carrying a light load on the level.

Grade 1: Light. Becomes short of breath with light activities such as walking on the level, washing, or standing.

Grade 0: No task. Becomes short of breath at rest, while sitting, or lying down.

W: Amount uncertain. Patient's ability to perform tasks is impaired due to shortness of breath, but amount cannot be specified. Details are not sufficient to allow impairment to be categorized.

X: Unknown. Information unavailable regarding limitation of magnitude of task.

Y: Impaired for reasons other than shortness of breath. For example, musculoskeletal problems or chest pain.

Magnitude of Effort

Grade 4: Extraordinary. Becomes short of breath only with the greatest imaginable effort. No shortness of breath with ordinary effort.

Grade 3: Major. Becomes short of breath with effort distinctly submaximal, but of major proportion. Tasks performed without pause unless the task requires extraordinary effort that may be performed with pause.

Grade 2: Moderate. Becomes short of breath with moderate effort. Tasks performed with occasional pauses and requiring longer to complete than the average person.

Grade 1: Light. Becomes short of breath with little effort. Tasks performed with little effort or more difficult tasks performed with frequent pauses and requiring 50% to 100% longer to complete than the average person might require.

Grade 0: No effort. Becomes short of breath at rest, while sitting, or lying down.

W: Amount uncertain. Patient's exertional ability is impaired due to shortness of breath, but amount cannot be specified. Details are not sufficient to allow impairment to be categorized.

X: Unknown. Information unavailable regarding limitations of effort.

Y: Impaired for reasons other than shortness of breath. For example, musculoskeletal problems or chest pain.

TRANSITIONAL DYSPNEA INDEX

Change in Functional Impairment

3: Major deterioration. Formerly working and has had to stop working and has completely abandoned some of usual activities due to shortness of breath.

2: Moderate. Deterioration. Formerly working and has had to stop working or has completely abandoned some of usual activities due to shortness of breath.

1: Minor deterioration. Has changed to a lighter job and/or has reduced activities in number or duration due to shortness of breath. Any deterioration less than proceeding categories.

0: No change. No change in functional status due to shortness of breath.

+1: Minor improvement. Able to return to work at reduced pace or has resumed some customary activities with more vigor than previously because of improvement in shortness of breath.

+2: Moderate improvement. Able to return to work at nearly usual pace and/or able to return to most activities with moderate restrictions only.

+3: Major improvement. Able to return to work at former pace and able to return to full activities with only mild restriction because of improvement of shortness of breath.

Z: Further impairment for reasons other than shortness of breath. Patient has stopped working, reduced work, or has given up or reduced other activities for other reasons. For example, other medical problems, being "laid off" from work, and so forth.

Change in Magnitude of Task

−3: Major deterioration. Has deteriorated two grades or greater from baseline status.

−2: Moderate deterioration. Has deterioration at least one grade, but fewer than two grades from baseline status.

−1: Minor deterioration. Has deteriorated less than one grade from baseline. Patient with distinct deterioration within grade, but has not changed grades.

0: No changes. No change from baseline.

+1: Minor improvement. Has improved less than one grade from baseline. Patient with distinct improvement with grade, but has not changed grades.

+2: Moderate improvement. Has improved at least one grade, but fewer than two grades from baseline.

+3: Major improvement. Has improved two grades or greater from baseline.

Z: Further impairment for reasons other than shortness of breath. Patient has reduced exertional capacity, but not related to shortness of breath—for example, musculoskeletal problems or chest pain.

Changes in Magnitude of Effort

−3: Major deterioration. Severe decrease in effort from baseline to avoid shortness of breath. Activities now take 50% to 100% longer to complete than required at baseline.

−2: Moderate deterioration. Some decreases in effort to avoid shortness of breath, although not as great as preceding category. There is greater pausing with some activities.

−1: Minor deterioration. Does not require more pause to avoid shortness of breath, but does things with distinctly less effort than previously to avoid breathlessness.

0: No change. No change in effort to avoid shortness of breath.

+1: Minor improvement. Able to do things with distinctly greater effort without shortness of breath. For example, may be able to carry out tasks somewhat more rapidly than previously.

+2: Moderate improvement. Able to do things with fewer pauses and distinctly greater effort without shortness of breath. Improvement is greater than proceeding category, but not of major proportion.

+3: Major improvement. Able to do things with much greater effort than previously with few, if any, pauses. For example, activities may be performed 50% to 100% more rapidly than at baseline.

Z: Further impairment for reasons other than shortness of breath. Patient has reduced exertional capacity, but not related to shortness of breath. For example, musculoskeletal problems or chest pains.

Mahler DA, Weinberg DH, Wells CK, Feinstein AR. The measurement of dyspnea. Contents, interobserver agreement, and physiologic correlates of two new clinical indexes. *Chest* 1984;85:751–758.

CHAPTER 6

Pulmonary Function and Respiratory Assessment of Neuromuscular Patients: Objective Measures of Lung Function

CHAPTER OUTLINE

Clinical Uses of PFT
MIP
   Definition
   Methods of Measurement
   Interpretation
MEP
   Definition
   Methods of Measurement
   Interpretation
PCF
   Definition
   Methods of Measurement
   Interpretation
Sniff Nasal Inspiratory Pressure Test
   Definition
   Methods of Measurement
   Interpretation
Other Measures of Pulmonary Function
   Maximum Voluntary Ventilation
   Tension Time Index (P_{100})
   Transdiaphragmatic Pressure (P_{di})
   Supine Pulmonary Function Tests
Noninvasive Measures of Pulmonary Function
   Pulse Oximetry
   Capnography
Monitoring of Respiratory Function During Sleep
   Polysomnography
   Nocturnal Pulse Oximetry
   Nocturnal Capnography
Laboratory Measures
   Serum Bicarbonate and Chloride
   Arterial Blood Gases
Summary
References
Questions for Research

INTRODUCTION

The purpose of a thorough pulmonary evaluation of patients with amyotrophic lateral sclerosis (ALS) is to determine the degree of respiratory impairment and track its course. Respiratory muscle strength, as measured by vital capacity (VC), maximum inspiratory pressure (MIP), and maximum expiratory pressure (MEP), is an important prognostic factor in ALS (Lyall et al., 2001). Baseline pulmonary function testing (PFT) should be performed on the initial visit to the neuromuscular clinic and should be repeated on each subsequent visit (Miller et al., 1999). A detailed respiratory assessment should be conducted during each quarterly clinic visit. The initial respiratory assessment should include the following:

- Clinical assessment and signs of respiratory insufficiency
- Sleep quality and symptoms of nocturnal hypoventilation
- Upper airway function
- Past medical history and co-morbidities
- Risk assessment for pulmonary and cardiovascular complications

This chapter covers pulmonary function tests and their diagnostic significance in ALS. It also includes useful laboratory tests and measures of gas exchange.

MEASURES OF LUNG MECHANICS AND STRENGTH

In the clinic setting, VC, inspiratory and expiratory flow rates, and inspiratory pressures allow respiratory care practitioners to categorize a respiratory abnormality, monitor progression of respiratory muscle weakness, and determine the need for and timing of treatment. Serial measurements of pulmonary function tests are recommended in the management of ALS (Heffernan et al., 2006). In the United States, PFT results are used to determine insurance reimbursement for respiratory assistive devices and acceptance into hospice care. Forced VC (FVC) is the most commonly used measure of lung function in ALS clinics (Melo et al., 1999). It is a significant predictor of survival in ALS (Czaplinski et al., 2006; Haverkamp et al., 1995). It is included in the standards adopted by the

American Academy of Neurology in its ALS Practice Parameters (Miller et al., 1999). FVC is used as a guideline when assessing patient risk during invasive procedures, such as percutaneous endoscopic gastrostomy (PEG) and as inclusion criteria for research studies. Simple spirometry measures are obtained in outpatient clinics using handheld devices that yield valid and reproducible results (Barr et al., 2008).

For the primary tests of pulmonary mechanics and function, we include the following:

- Definition
- Method of measurement
- Interpretation or diagnostic significance

SPIROMETRY

Definition

Spirometry is a pulmonary function test that measures volume and flow of inhaled and exhaled gases. In the clinic setting, portable spirometers are used to record the flow of air and volumes over time. Actual values of the patient are plotted in a graphic display and compared with normal values in healthy people of the same age, height, and gender and are displayed as a percentage of the two. Office-based spirometry focuses primarily on VC (expressed in liters) exhaled forcefully after a maximum inhalation (FVC), lung volumes exhaled in 1 second after a maximum inhalation (FEV$_1$), and the ratio of the two (FEV$_1$/FVC).

Most office-based spirometers are handheld devices that consist of a microcomputer, flow sensor, and disposable mouthpiece. Values are displayed on a liquid crystal display screen. Spirometers have data storage capability and can be attached to a printer. These handheld devices produce good quality spirometry and accurate interpretation (Yawn et al., 2007).

VITAL CAPACITY (VC)

Definition

VC is the maximal volume of air exhaled from the point of maximal inhalation. This is considered a "slow" VC and is measured in liters. FVC measures the maximum volume of air that can be forcefully exhaled following a maximum inhalation, a volume displacement technique.

Methods of Measurement

Spirometry is performed with patients in a sitting position. Mouthpiece and nose clips are used. In the case of lip weakness, in which a patient may not be able to maintain a tight seal around the mouthpiece, a mask will be used. Patients are instructed to breathe normally and then inhale quickly to maximum volume and immediately exhale rapidly until the lungs are empty. Accurate spirometry results are dependent on the cooperation of the patient, their ability to understand and follow instruction, and the training and skill of the person conducting the test. Consistency in patient instruction, expiratory technique, and spirometer are necessary when monitoring changes over time. Ideally, the same person will measure pulmonary function during each clinic visit.

The American Thoracic Society recommends that three reproducible tests be obtained. In a reproducible test, FVC and FEV_1 will not vary more than 5%.

Acceptable spirometry will include the following:

- Minimal delay from start of inhalation to initiation of forceful exhalation
- Patient is free of cough for the first second
- Patient has good glottic function
- Complete exhalation (at least 6 seconds)
- No leakage around mouthpiece or mask
- No obstruction of mouthpiece by patient's tongue

For patents with bulbar muscle weakness who may experience partial upper airway obstruction during forceful expiratory maneuvers, a slow VC can be used. In a slow VC, the patient inhales to maximum volume and exhales slowly but completely until the lungs are empty.

Interpretation

A loss of respiratory muscle innervation leads to restrictive pulmonary disease, evidenced by stiffening of the lungs, decreased ability to inhale fully, and loss of volume. Changes in VC do not identify weakness in specific respiratory muscles. Although VC is reduced by pulmonary muscle weakness, it also reflects changes in lung parenchyma, chest wall, alveoli and airways (Lechtzin 2006). VC may not be significantly reduced until respiratory muscle strength is less than 50% of normal (Rochester & Esau, 1994). Progression of respiratory muscle weakness is evaluated by the rate of decline of VC (Czaplinski et al., 2006). Current American Academy of Neurology practice parameters includes routine assessment of upright FVC to measure respiratory muscle function (Miller et al., 1999).

EXPIRATORY VOLUME

Definition

The volume of air that can be expelled during the first second of the forced exhalation maneuver is the forced expiratory volume (FEV_1). It is a measure of the rate of flow of exhaled air and expressed in liters.

Methods of Measurement

Forced expiratory volumes are obtained as part of the FVC described previously.

Interpretation

A decrease in lung expansion results in decreased elastic recoil on exhalation. This brings a concomitant reduction in FEV_1; therefore, the ratio of VC and expiratory volume (FEV_1/FVC) is usually within normal limits, a classic restrictive picture. This is seen in patients with neuromuscular disease, sarcoidosis, intersitial fibrosis, and chest wall deformities. FEV_1 may be further reduced in patients with poorly controlled reactive airway disease (asthma), vocal cord dysfunction, or those prone to airway collapse on exhalation (emphysema). Although total lung capacity (TLC) is decreased in restrictive disease, functional residual capacity (FRC) may remain within normal limits. Expiratory muscle weakness will result in an increase in residual volume (RV).

Graphic displays of inspiratory and expiratory flow rates assist the clinician in interpreting numerical results. Upper-airway obstruction, seen in patients with moderate-to-severe bulbar muscle weakness, results in a "sawtooth" pattern on exhalation. Upper-airway closure on inhalation is seen as an indentation or notch on a flow-volume loop.

CLINICAL USES OF PFT

- FVC < 80% of predicted and FEV_1 < 80% of predicted with a normal FEV_1/FVC ratio indicate the presence of restrictive lung disease.
- The average decline of VC in ALS is 2.3% per month and follows a linear course (Schiffman & Belsh, 1993).
- Median survival of patients with ALS with baseline FVC < 75% at diagnosis has been shown to be 2.91 years, compared with 4.08 years with baseline > 75% (Czaplinski et al., 2006).
- Because FVC has been shown to predict survival and disease progression in ALS, it is useful as an inclusion or exclusion criterion for clinical trials (Brinkman et al., 1997; Czaplinski et al., 2006).
- Postoperative risk with PEG increases when FVC declines below 50% of predicted (Kasarskis et al., 1999).
- Normal VC is 60 to 70 mL/kg of ideal body weight. Patients whose VC drops below 30 mL/kg will experience decreased expiratory flow rates, weak cough, impaired secretion clearance, and risk of atelectasis (Bella & Chad, 1998; Mehta, 2006).
- If a patient's VC falls to 15 mL/kg or 1 L, he or she is considered to be in acute respiratory failure. Continuous ventilation, invasively or noninvasively, is usually required at this point (Mehta, 2006).
- FVC of ≤ 30% of predicted is used as an admission criterion for hospice care.

MIP

Definition

The amount of negative pressure a patient can exert on inhalation against an occluded airway is referred to as MIP, negative inspiratory force or PI_{max}. MIP is an isometric maneuver and a sensitive test of global inspiratory muscle strength. Decreases in MIP values may therefore be more sensitive to respiratory decline and better correlate with symptoms in patients with neuromuscular disease than FVC.

Methods of Measurement

MIP is a static (no flow) maneuver in which the patient exhales to RV and then quickly and forcefully inhales as the technician briefly occludes the airway for at least 1 second. In the outpatient setting, MIP can be performed using a portable handheld device with electronic pressure transducer or a manometer. Mouthpiece or mask may be used. In patients with bulbar muscle denervation, mouth weakness may make this test difficult to perform. In addition, one can generate negative pressure with mouth muscles against a closed glottis when a tapered mouthpiece is used. In these instances, it is preferable to use a disposable oronasal mask to obtain accurate values. A small leak at the distal end of the MIP device may prevent the facial muscles from generating significant pressures and affecting results.

The manufacturer of a handheld respiratory pressure meter with micro-computer (MicroRPM, Micro Medical Ltd., Chatham, Kent, UK) recommends exhalation to RV; however, others recommend MIP be measured from FRC because inspiratory muscle strength is overestimated at levels below FRC because of elastic recoil pressure of the thorax (Uldry & Fitting, 1995). Consistency in technique and instruction is the most important factor in tracking changes in inspiratory muscle strength and lung function decline.

Interpretation

Adequate inspiratory pressures are necessary to maintain normal ventilation and gas exchange.

MIP is usually expressed as an absolute number as there is a wide range of predictive values and nomograms have yet to be validated. Low values have been shown to correlate with nocturnal oxygen desaturation (David et al., 1997).

Normal MIP is considered to be ≤ -90 cm H_2O to ≤ -120 cm H_2O, with men in the upper range and women at the lower. In some pulmonary function laboratories -108 cm H_2O is used as a reference value to which actual patient values are compared. In the United States, > -60 cm H_2O is considered by the Centers for Medicare and Medicaid Services to be an indication for the need for assisted ventilation. Values > -30 cm H_2O are associated with progression to respiratory failure (Mehta, 2006). Again, MIP may be a more sensitive measure of respiratory insufficiency than FVC in ALS; however, it may be that under current Centers for Medicare and Medicaid Services guidelines patients more easily qualify for respiratory assistive devices using MIP values than those for FVC.

MEP

Definition

MEP or PE_{max} measures the strength of the expiratory muscles (the internal intercostals and abdominals).

Methods of Measurement

MEP may also be performed in a pulmonary function laboratory or outpatient clinic using a handheld pressure transducer or manometer as described for MIP. MEP is a static maneuver performed against an occluded airway. The technique for obtaining MEP follows the same guidelines as MIP, with MEP measured from TLC. Peak cough expiratory flow, also known as peak cough flow (PCF), measures may be obtained instead of, or in addition to, MEP to assess a patient's ability to clear pulmonary secretions.

Interpretation

Weak expiratory muscles lead to impaired cough and the inability to mobilize pulmonary secretions. Values are generally expressed as absolute values. Patients with neuromuscular disease should have MIP and MEP values measured serially to monitor respiratory muscle decline.

The technique for obtaining MIP and MEP in the outpatient clinic setting is as follows:

- MIP and MEP are measured with the patient in a seated position.
- Patients should be instructed to keep their shoulders, upper body, and abdominal muscles relaxed to allow for the natural downward movement of the diaphragm during inhalation.
- Restrictive clothing should be loosened, if necessary.
- If using mask, check for a proper fit so air leaks can be avoided.
- If using mouthpiece, make sure patient can maintain a tight seal. Use nose clips to prevent air leaks.
- Measure MIP from FRC. Measure MEP from TLC.
- Maintain static pressure for 2 seconds.
- Repeat three times or until two identical readings are obtained (Hart et al., 2003).
- Record the best measure obtained when a plateau is reached (two values of less than 10% difference) or when no more learning effect is seen (Volianitis et al., 2001).

PCF

Definition

PCF or peak cough flow is a simple yet valuable method of measuring a patient's ability to generate enough expiratory force to protect the lungs from inadvertent aspiration of food, liquid, or saliva.

Methods of Measurement

PCF is measured by using a cylindrical peak flow meter attached to a disposable oronasal mask. The patient is requested to take a deep breath and cough into the mask, moving the indicator up the cylinder to measure flow in liters per minute (LPM). RCPs will be familiar with this maneuver, as peak flow meters are used routinely to detect airway obstruction in patients with asthma.

Interpretation

A strong cough is necessary to clear pulmonary secretions. It is dependent on strong inspiratory and expiratory muscles and intact glottic function. PCF will be decreased if a patient cannot generate an FVC > 1.5 L.

Studies of PCF in patients with Duchenne muscular dystrophy are instructive, although the suggestions for treatment have not been validated. In one study, a flow rate of 270 LPM indicated high risk for retained secretions and need for mechanically assisted cough. PCF of 160 LPM was linked with greater risk of respiratory failure and need for intermittent noninvasive respiratory support. Tracheostomy was recommended if needed for pulmonary secretion clearance (Bach, 2002). Patients with ALS able to maintain a mean PCF above 337 LPM have been shown to have a significantly greater chance of being alive at 18 months after diagnosis (Chaudri et al., 2002).

Volume expansion using a manual resuscitation bag can increase PCF for a time immediately after administration. For those with weak expiratory muscles, mechanically assisted cough may be of assistance. A mechanical insufflator-exsufflator (MI-E), sold in the United States as the Cough Assist (Respironics, Murrysville, PA), is used to expand the lungs through positive pressure and evacuates the airways through negative pressure. If prescribed early in the disease course, it can be used to prevent retained secretions and reduce risk of pneumonia. Familiarity with this device enables patients to use it for secretion removal if acute infection develops. Lung expansion and secretion management techniques will be covered in greater detail in Chapter 7.

SNIFF NASAL INSPIRATORY PRESSURE TEST

Definition

Sniff nasal inspiratory pressure (SNIP) is one of the newer measures of inspiratory muscle strength. Used first in Europe, it has made its way to the United States but is not yet widely used. SNIP is a reliable noninvasive measure of global inspiratory muscle strength (Uldry & Fitting, 1995) and correlates with P_{di} (Morgan et al., 2005). It can be used when bulbar and facial muscle weaknesses preclude the use of MIP maneuver.

Methods of Measurement

A cylindrical nasal probe is inserted in one nostril. A good seal is necessary. The nasal probes are available in multiple sizes and the patient should be fitted prior to testing. The patient maximally "sniffs" (quickly breathes in through the nose) while a transducer records the pressure. The maneuver is usually performed with the contralateral (opposite) nostril open. Ten maneuvers are common, with the maximum value recorded. Rest periods of 30 seconds between sniffs are adequate to avoid fatigue.

Interpretation

Like MIP, SNIP is more sensitive to decreases in respiratory muscle strength than FVC (Lyall et al., 2001). SNIP correlates closely with P_{di}. Values of < 40 cm H_2O predicts mortality within 6 months (Morgan et al., 2005). In the absence of neuromuscular or lung disease, the mean normal value is 90 cm H_2O. SNIP values negatively correlate with age and are independent of height, body mass index, and gender (Uldry & Fitting, 1995). Although a close correlation between MIP and SNIP has been found, there is relatively poor agreement, especially in severe restrictive disease (Hart et al., 2003). MIP and SNIP probably reflect different aspects of inspiratory muscle function, with MIP measuring force and SNIP measuring pressure. MIP and SNIP should, therefore, be used as complementary methods of testing.

OTHER MEASURES OF PULMONARY FUNCTION

Maximum Voluntary Ventilation

Although not routinely performed in the outpatient clinic setting, maximum voluntary ventilation tests may be used to assess the fatigue of respiratory muscles during rapid, forceful breathing. This test appears to be more sensitive to pulmonary muscle weakness and respiratory decline than FVC; however, maximum voluntary ventilation is a tiring maneuver to perform, requires a maximum sustained effort, and is therefore difficult to reproduce during the pulmonary function test. Its usefulness in ALS has not been established.

Tension Time Index (P_{100})

The tension time index (TTI), also referred to as the pressure time index, is a measure of the *work being done* by the diaphragm and diaphragmatic fatigue. It is a novel noninvasive measurement used almost exclusively in pulmonary research. It is obtained during normal tidal volume breathing in the course of PFT in the laboratory setting. During the inspiratory phase, pressures are recorded during a passive 0.1-second static maneuver. The index is calculated by comparing the inspiratory time with the total time. Unlike transdiaphragmatic pressure tests (P_{di}), the TTI gives a comparatively accurate assessment of diaphragm strength without the discomfort of an invasive procedure. In patients with moderate-to-severe bulbar muscle involvement, it may be better tolerated and produce more accurate results than forced inspiratory and expiratory maneuvers.

Transdiaphragmatic Pressure (P_{di})

P_{di} is the "gold standard" of patient-independent tests to which non-invasive, volitional tests of diaphragm muscle strength are compared (Miller et al., 1985). Transdiaphragmatic pressures are obtained by inserting balloons into the stomach and midesophagus and measuring the pressure difference across the diaphragm while the patient performs a maximal sniff maneuver. It is uncomfortable and patients may not tolerate the test. P_{di} is used most frequently in research studies (Lechtzin, 2006). Presently, noninvasive measures of diaphragm muscle strength that can be performed routinely in a physician's office, pulmonary function laboratory, or multidisciplinary ALS clinic are preferable.

Supine Pulmonary Function Tests

Performing pulmonary function tests with the patient lying flat on his or her back is a better predictor of diaphragm muscle weakness than those performed in the seated or standing position (Varrato et al., 2001). Supine FVC values correlate positively with P_{di} lending it credibility in the measurement of diaphragm weakness. In patients with neuromuscular disease, the difference in upright versus supine FVC is greater than for those with normal lungs (> 25% change versus < 10%) (Fromageot et al., 2001). Supine FVC and supine MIP should be performed if patients report symptoms of nocturnal hypoventilation when upright spirometry values are within normal limits (Lechtzin et al., 2002).

NONINVASIVE MEASURES OF LUNG FUNCTION

Pulse Oximetry

Definition

Ninety-eight percent of oxygen molecules in the blood are bound to hemoglobin, circulate in the arterial vessels, and then are delivered to the tissues. Since the 1990s, pulse oximetry has been widely accepted as the primary noninvasive method of monitoring oxygenation. Pulse oximetry measures oxyhemoglobin saturation through light absorption across an arterial tissue bed of finger, toe, or earlobe.

Method of Measurements

Through the use of red and infrared light emitting diodes and measurement of light absorption across a pulsatile blood vessel, oximeters are able to measure the amount of arterial hemoglobin saturated with oxygen molecules. Accuracy of pulse oximetry is generally ± 4% of actual values when saturations are above 70%.

Interpretation

In the early stages of ALS, diurnal resting oximetry is not sensitive in predicting decline in respiratory function. The shape of the oxyhemoglobin dissociation curve assures that $PaCO_2$ can increase significantly before there is evidence of oxygen desaturation due to oxygen molecule unloading at the tissue sites; therefore, SpO_2 may decline only in the late stages of the disease. In a study of indications for tracheostomy in ALS, daytime SpO_2 below 95% that could not be improved with the use of noninvasive ventilation was correlated with a likelihood of death or tracheostomy within 2 months (Bach et al., 2004).

Clinicians should be suspicious if patients present with elevated heart rate and respiratory rate, as these may be responses to compromised gas exchange. Chronic hypoxemia results in pulmonary vasoconstriction, vascular resistance, and risk of right-sided heart failure.

Capnography

Definition

Capnography analyzes the change in concentration of CO_2 in exhaled gas over time. The results are displayed as partial pressure or percentage (capnometry) or in concentration of CO_2 over time (capnogram).

Methods of Measurement

Analyzing CO_2 in a nonintubated, spontaneously breathing patient is achieved by sampling gas from a patient's airway. Side-stream CO_2 collectors sample exhaled gas continuously where it is detected; results are displayed graphically and numerically. Recent improvements in this technology have reduced or eliminated measurement limitations of the past, lag time between sampling and display of values, blockage of sample tubing by mucus, or contamination of the detector with moisture. Data storage capabilities allow patients to use portable end-tidal CO_2 monitors at home during sleep; however, the accuracy of these new capnography units, especially in the face of anatomical dead space ventilation (caused by hyperventilation), has yet to be verified.

Interpretation

As the diaphragm, intercostals, abdominals, and other muscles of respiration continue to lose innervation, they become weakened and fatigued. Significant fatigue occurs when pressures needed to generate normal resting tidal volumes exceed the maximum pressure respiratory muscles can generate (Schiffman, 1996). Elevated end-tidal CO_2 (ETCO$_2$) occurs with hypercapnia in spontaneously breathing patients. Daytime hypercapnia as an indicator of hypoventilation in ALS has yet to be studied but it has the potential for detecting early respiratory insufficiency.

ETCO$_2$ monitoring correlates well with PaCO$_2$ in the absence of lung or cardiovascular disease (Morley et al., 1993).

MONITORING OF RESPIRATORY FUNCTION DURING SLEEP

Polysomnography

Polysomnography may be needed in a small number of ALS patients. Patient-reported symptoms of nocturnal hypoventilation and sleep disordered breathing in the absence of objective measures of respiratory muscle decline can be assessed with polysomnography, or sleep study. Studies have shown obstructive and central apneas in patients with ALS (Arnulf et al., 2000); however, there is a great deal of variability in studies of nocturnal respiratory insufficiency in ALS (Lyall et al., 2001).

Patients can be evaluated by a sleep technologist in the laboratory setting or by use of an ambulatory device used at home, with data extracted and interpreted at a later time. In the laboratory setting, the number of "arousals" is recorded. An arousal is defined as movement from a deep, restorative level of sleep to a lighter level of sleep, although not necessarily into wakefulness. The arousal periods are usually precipitated by hypopneas or apneas of such severity and duration that oxygenation desaturation occurs. The desaturation causes the body to move from a deep sleep into a lighter stage, enabling the patient to breathe more deeply, normalizing oxygen levels. All events during the sleep period are recorded with the total number of apneas and hypopneas combined and summarized as the apnea-hypopnea index, or number of events per hour. More than 5 events per hour are defined as abnormal. A desaturation event can be defined as a 4% change from baseline or a drop below 90% for 2 cumulative minutes (Jackson et al., 2001).

Obstructive apnea in ALS is atypical, but hypoventilation is common as the diaphragm weakens, leading to nocturnal oxygen desaturation and hypercapnia. Patients with ALS may complain of waking in the morning tired or not refreshed despite having slept for a full 8 to 9 hours. In rapid eye movement (REM) sleep, the stage required for physical and emotional health, all muscles in the body are essentially immobilized except for the diaphragm and ocular muscles. Because the accessory muscles cannot be of assistance in the event of diaphragmatic weakness, the body will compromise by arousing the patient from REM sleep into a lighter level, allowing other muscles to assist in lung expansion. Homeostasis will triumph at the expense of a good night's sleep. Detailed questioning by clinicians may elicit symptoms of obstructive sleep apnea that existed before a diagnosis of ALS.

Nocturnal Pulse Oximetry

Nocturnal hypoventilation is one of the earliest indicators of respiratory insufficiency in ALS. It may occur before daytime clinical symptoms are reported (Heffernan et al., 2006). Nocturnal pulse oximetry is a less extensive but less expensive alternative to polysomnography for monitoring respiratory function during sleep. It may be used as a screening tool to suggest the need for a more detailed sleep study. Small portable oximeters can store data to be downloaded and analyzed at a later time. Patients may be sleeping poorly for a number of other reasons (muscle spasms, discomfort, depression, and anxiety among them), and physicians should explore these possibilities and offer treatment.

Nocturnal Capnography

Portable capnography devices to measure $ETCO_2$ in the home are now available (LifeSense, Nonin Medical, Plymouth, MN). Combination oximetry/capnography units use side-stream flow and store data overnight to be downloaded and interpreted at a later time. If able to be accurately recorded at night, $ETCO_2$ could serve as a sensitive test of respiratory insufficiency as hypercapnia during sleep is an early sign of ventilatory failure. A drawback of the current technology is its inability to capture dead space ventilation, often seen in patients with chronic respiratory insufficiency, in the digital $ETCO_2$ readout data. Home-based nocturnal $ETCO_2$ monitoring in ALS has yet to be studied.

LABORATORY MEASURES

Serum Bicarbonate and Chloride

Small studies have shown a correlation between respiratory symptoms and elevated serum bicarbonate (HCO_3^-) and decreased serum chloride (Cl^-)

levels. These laboratory measures are especially useful in patients with severe bulbar involvement whose pulmonary function cannot be accurately measured or at the end stage of the disease (Hadjikoutis, 2001). Serum chloride reflects the degree of respiratory acidosis. Elevated serum bicarbonate is seen with chronic hypercapnia. HCO_3^- exists first as CO_2 and then as carbonic acid, H_2CO_3. Bicarbonate, which is regulated by the kidneys, is the major extracellular buffer in the blood. These laboratory findings are consistent with compensated respiratory acidosis, a situation in which the kidney reabsorbs bicarbonate in response to increased hydrogen ion (H^+) secretion.

Arterial Blood Gases

Arterial blood gas measures are not used for routine screening in ALS. Daytime oxygen levels are rarely reduced until very late in the disease process. With mild weakness, PCO_2 falls bellow normal as hyperventilation compensates for alveolar hypoxemia (Lyall et al., 2001). Hypercapnia first develops nocturnally because of hypoventilation in REM sleep. Diurnal hypercapnia does not develop until respiratory muscle weakness is quite advanced (Rochester & Esau, 1994); therefore, oxygen and carbon dioxide do not appear to have predictive power in ALS progression. A longitudinal study of pulmonary predictors of survival in ALS did not find a significant association between $PaCO_2$ and longevity in the 95 patients followed (Schmidt et al., 2006).

Clinical observation and anecdote point to a subset of ALS patients who are able to maintain FVC above 50% of predicted without reports of significant respiratory discomfort who develop compensated respiratory acidosis. These may be patients who have been able to use accessory muscles in the face of moderate-to-severe diaphragmatic weakness. If chronically elevated $PaCO_2$ is suspected, these patients should be closely monitored, as they could acutely decompensate if they contract a respiratory infection or develop mucus plugging. Because of a lack of respiratory reserve, they are at risk for acute respiratory failure. In this event, patients could face emergency intubation and ventilation, a situation the majority of people with ALS elect against. Patients with chronic hypercapnia should be warned that the administration of supplemental oxygen can be detrimental by blunting ventilatory drive, contributing to atelectasis and leading to acute respiratory failure. A "MediAlert" bracelet, worn by the patient, can warn emergency medical technicians and emergency department staff that decreased SpO_2 levels should not be treated with oxygen.

SUMMARY

The majority of the measures of lung mechanics described previously here are volitional, meaning they are dependent on the patient's effort, cooperation, and understanding of what is expected. Patients whose bulbar muscles are impaired may have difficulty performing effort-dependent respiratory tests. Lung function values that do not correspond to patient-reported symptoms of hypoventilation may be difficult to interpret. There is no evidence informing us which is the best test for detecting early signs of impending respiratory failure (Miller et al., 1999) or at what level of respiratory muscle weakness hypoventilation occurs (Lyall et al., 2001). RCPs are encouraged to pursue correlations between subjective symptoms of respiratory insufficiency, standard pulmonary function measures, and novel measures, such as TTI. This will aid clinicians in determining the most sensitive measures of respiratory insufficiency and the timing of intervention.

REFERENCES

Amulf I, Similowski T, Salachas F, Garma C, Mehiri S, Attali V. Sleep disorders and diaphragm function in patients with amyotrophic lateral sclerosis. *Am J Respir Crit Care Med* 2000;161(3 Pt 1):849–856.

Bach JR. Amyotrophic lateral sclerosis: prolongation of life by noninvasive respiratory aids. *Chest* 2002;122:92–98.

Bach JR, Bianchi C, Aufiero E. Oximetry and indications for tracheostomy for amyotrophic lateral sclerosis. *Chest* 2004;126:1502–1507.

Barr RG, Stemple KJ, Mesia-Vela S, et al. Reproducibility and validity of a handheld spirometer. *Respiratory Care* 2008;53:433–441.

Bella I, Chad DA. Neuromuscular disorders and acute respiratory failure. *Neurol Clin* 1998;16:391–417.

Brinkman JR, Mendoza M, Andres P, et al. Guidelines for the use and performance of quantitative outcome measures in ALS clinical trials. *J Neurol Sci* 1997;147: 97–111.

Chaudri MB, Liu C, Hubbard R, Jefferson D, Kinnear WJ. Relationship between supramaximal flow during cough and mortality in motor neuron disease. *Eur Respir J* 2002:19:434–438.

Czaplinski A, Yen AA, Appel SH. Forced vital capacity (FVC) as an indicator of survival and disease progression in an ALS clinic population. *J Neurol Neurosurg Psychiatry* 2006;77:390–392.

David WS, Bundlie SR, Mahdavi Z. Polysomnographic studies in amyotrophic lateral sclerosis. *J Neurol Sci* 1997;153(Suppl 1):S29–S35.

Fromageot C, Lofaso F, Annane D, et al. Supine fall in lung volumes in the assessment of diaphragmatic weakness in neuromuscular disorders. *Arch Phys Med Rehab* 2001;82:123–128.

Hart N, Polkey MI, Sharshar T, et al. Limits of sniff nasal pressure in patients with severe neuromuscular weakness. *J Neurol Neurosurg Psych* 2003;74:1685–1687.

Haverkamp LJ, Appel V, Appel SH. Natural history of amyotrophic lateral sclerosis in a database population: validation of a scoring system and a model for survival prediction. *Brain* 1995;118:707–719.

Heffernan C, Jenkinson C, Holmes T, et al. Management of respiration in MND/ALS patients: an evidence based review. *Amyotrophic Lateral Sclerosis* 2006; 7:5–15.

Jackson CE, Rosenfeld J, Moore DH, et al. A preliminary evaluation of a prospective study of pulmonary function studies and symptoms of hypoventilation in MND/ALS patients. *J Neurol Sci* 2001;191:75–78.

Kasarskis EJ, Scarlata D, Hill R, Fuller C, Stambler N, Cedarbaum JM. A retrospective study of percutaneous endoscopic gastrostomy in ALS patients during BDNF and CNTF trials. *J Neurol Sci* 1999;169:118–125.

Lechtzin N. Respiratory effects of amyotrophic lateral sclerosis: problems and solutions. *Respir Care* 2006;51:871–881.

Lechtzin N, Wiener CM, Shade DM, Clawson L, Diette GB. Spirometry in the supine position improves the detection of diaphragmatic weakness in patients with amyotrophic lateral sclerosis. *Chest* 2002;121:436–442.

Lyall RA, Donaldson N, Polkey ML, Leigh PN, Moxham J. Respiratory muscle strength and ventilatory failure in amyotrophic lateral sclerosis. *Brain* 2001;24: 2000–2013.

Mehta S. Neuromuscular disease causing acute respiratory failure. *Respir Care* 2006;51:1016–1023.

Melo, J, Homma A, Iturriaga E, et al. Pulmonary evaluation and prevalence of non-invasive ventilation in patients with amyotrophic lateral sclerosis: a multicenter survey and proposal of a pulmonary protocol. *J Neurol Sci* 1999;169:114–117.

Miller JM, Moxham J, Green M. The maximal sniff in the assessment of diaphragm function in man. *Clin Sci (Lond)* 1985;69:91–96.

Miller RG, Rosenberg JA, Gelinas DF, et al. Practice parameter: the care of the patient with amyotrophic lateral sclerosis (an evidence-based review): report of the Quality Standards Subcommittee of the American Academy of Neurology: ALS Practice Parameters Task Force. *Neurology* 1999;52:1311–1323.

Morgan RK, McNally S, Alexander M, Conroy R, Haediman O, Costello RW. Use of sniff nasal-inspiratory force to predict survival in amyotrophic lateral sclerosis. *Am J Crit Care Med* 2005;171:269–274.

Morley TF, Giaimo J, Maroszan E, et al. Use of capnography for assessment of the adequacy of alveolar ventilation during the weaning from mechanical ventilation. *Am Rev Respir Dis* 1993;148:339–344.

Rochester DF, Esau SA. Assessment of ventilatory function in patients with neuro-muscular disease. *Clin Chest Med* 1994;15:751–763.

Schiffman PL. Pulmonary function and respiratory management of the ALS patient. In Belsh JM, Schiffman PL(eds.). *Amyotrophic Lateral Sclerosis: Diagnosis and Management for the Clinician.* Armonk, NY: Futura Publishing Co.; 1996, pp. 333–355.

Schiffman PL, Belsh JM. Pulmonary function at diagnosis of amyotrophic lateral sclerosis: rate of deterioration. *Chest* 1993;103:508–513.

Schmidt EP, Drachman DB, Wiener CM, Clawson L, Kimball R, Lechtzin N. Pulmonary predictors of survival in amyotrophic lateral sclerosis: use in clinical trial design. *Muscle Nerve* 2006;33:127–132.

Uldry C, Fitting JW. Maximal values of sniff nasal inspiratory pressure in health subjects. *Thorax* 1995;50:371–375.

Varrato J, Siderowf A, Damiano P, Gregory S, Feinberg D, McCluskey L. Postural change of forced vital capacity predicts some respiratory symptoms in ALS. *Neurology* 2001;57:357–359.

Volianitis S, McConnell AK, Jones DA. Assessment of maximum inspiratory pressure. *Respiration* 2001;68:22–27.

Yawn BP, Enright PL, Lemanske RF Jr, et al. Spirometry can be done in family physicians' offices and alters clinical decisions in management of asthma and COPD. *Chest* 2007;132:1162–1168.

QUESTIONS FOR RESEARCH

1. Which pulmonary function measures best predict respiratory muscle decline in ALS?

2. Which measures of lung function predict early respiratory insufficiency in ALS?

3. What are the earliest subjective symptoms of respiratory muscle weakness in ALS?

4. Which pulmonary function measures correlate with subjective symptoms of respiratory insufficiency in the early stages of ALS?

5. How effective are $ETCO_2$ monitors in detecting nocturnal hypoventilation in ALS?

Volume Expansion, Secretion Mobilization, and Cough Assistance in Amyotrophic Lateral Sclerosis

CHAPTER OUTLINE

INTRODUCTION

Respiratory failure in amyotrophic lateral sclerosis results from weakness in the major muscles of inspiration and expiration. Inspiratory muscle weakness leads to decreased ventilation that in turn leads to atelectasis and impaired gas exchange. Lower-extremity weakness leads to decreased mobility and exercise, reducing lung expansion and risk of retained secretions. Upper-airway muscle weakness leads to aspiration and bacterial contamination of the lower airway. Expiratory muscle weakness combined with glottic and inspiratory muscle weakness leads to an inability to cough and mobilize pulmonary secretions (Benditt, 2006a). Without intervention, patients with amyotrophic lateral sclerosis (ALS) are at risk of pneumonia and subsequent respiratory failure.

In multidisciplinary ALS clinics, respiratory care practitioners (RCPs) take a proactive approach to impaired ventilation, cough insufficiency, and airway clearance. Volume expansion, secretion mobilization, and assisted cough techniques are demonstrated and recommended. The goals of intervention are to maintain alveolar ventilation, optimize blood gases, increase cough flows, avoid hospitalization, and prevent acute respiratory failure due to pulmonary infection. Patients and family members can be educated about early signs and symptoms of respiratory infection. They are encouraged to contact their primary care physician or pulmonologist if they suspect infection so that assessment and treatment can be quickly initiated.

This chapter covers the techniques that are used to augment lung and chest wall expansion, secretion mobilization, and cough in patients with

ALS. Strong scientific evidence to support any airway clearance technique is lacking. Clinicians often rely on small studies, clinical observations, and expert opinion to guide choices. As no evidence-based guidelines exist, decisions on when and how to initiate treatment are empirically driven (Toussaint et al., 2006). Much of the published research on volume expansion techniques have been done with Duchenne muscular dystrophy (DMD) and spinal cord injury and benefits can only be inferred in ALS.

At the most basic level, it is unclear whether increased mucus production and airway secretions are a good thing or a bad thing. Before initiating therapy, RCPs should evaluate the pathophysiologic reasoning behind a secretion clearance technique (Hess, 2002). Treatment benefits and desired outcomes should be defined and therapy discontinued if these are not met. Given the lack of research on airway clearance in ALS, treatments will need to be individualized for each patient. The most useful outcome measure may be improved quality of life as defined by the patient, especially as palliation is the main goal of treatment in ALS.

PATIENT ASSESSMENT

Clinical respiratory assessment and pulmonary function have been covered in detail in Chapter 5 and are only briefly reviewed here. The palliative nature of care in ALS emphasizes symptom management and relief. Serial tests of pulmonary function, cough effectiveness, dyspnea, and clinical signs of hypoventilation all inform treatment recommendations.

Goals of lung volume recruitment in ALS:

To improve cough effectiveness
To improve voice function
To prevent microatelectasis
To improve pulmonary compliance
To decrease work of breathing
To assist spontaneous breathing during periods off NPPV
To improve quality of life

Adapted from Bach (2002a).

LUNG VOLUME RECRUITMENT

In ALS, respiratory impairment is demonstrated by reduction in vital capacity, expiratory flow rates, and lung compliance. Respiratory impairment may be inferred by a patient's soft voice and short sentences (due to low tidal volumes and decreased expiratory flow through the vocal cords). Reported signs include dyspnea with conversation and the inability to speak long sentences.

Incentive Spirometry

RCPs are familiar with incentive spirometry, also known as sustained maximal inspiration, as a method of preventing and treating postsurgical atelectasis in spontaneously breathing patients. Hand-held incentive spirometers have two indicators to assist in proper technique: (1) a volume indicator to measure lung volumes in liters and (2) a floating indictor used to visualize a steady and sustained inhalation. The goal is to generate a large inspiratory volume and a large distending pressure, followed by a breath hold of a few seconds.

Patients with lower-extremity onset ALS have reduced mobility and may use walkers or wheelchairs. Reduced activity may lead to microatelectasis and reduced oxygen levels and put patients at risk for pulmonary infection. Pulmonary muscle weakness may be slow to develop in this group, and patients will maintain their vital capacity capability. Deep breathing and breath-hold maneuvers with volume indicator are useful in recruiting underinflated alveoli. It gives patients an opportunity to actively participate in maintaining pulmonary health. A routine of 10 breaths two to three times a day followed each time by coughing to clear any mobilized secretions is recommended.

Manual Hyperinflation Therapy

Manual hyperinflation therapy, also called breath stacking or air stacking, is another method of preventing or treating atelectasis, providing transient improvement in lung and chest wall compliance, and assisting in cough augmentation (Lechtzin et al., 2006). After patients lose the ability spontaneously to inflate the lungs to maximum capacity, assistance is needed. Breath stacking is often the first respiratory assistive device used by patients with ALS. There are no specific guidelines for initiation of manual hyperinflation therapy. Bach (2002a) recommends initiating breath stacking before vital capacity drops to 70% of predicted values.

This low-tech method incorporates a self-inflating manual resuscitation bag, a one-way valve at the bag outlet port, corrugated tubing, and a plastic mouthpiece (Kang & Bach, 2000). If lip weakness prevents a seal or velum weakness allows for nasopharyngeal communication, a lip seal or oronasal face mask can be used. The technique involves using the resuscitation bag to inflate the lungs to maximum insufflation capacity. If the patient has adequate hand strength, breath stacking may be accomplished independently. Patients may also repeatedly compress the resuscitation bag by placing it between the upper arm and side of the chest or, with a longer circuit, using foot compression.

Maximum insufflation is achieved by having the patient take a deep breath then coordinating consecutive inhalations with brief compressions of the manual resuscitation bag with breath holding (through glottic closure) between each breath. A routine of 10 breaths two to three times a day is recommended. Cough strength can be augmented by breath stacking alone or in conjunction with abdominal compression (Trebbia et al., 2005). Breath stacking is well tolerated by most patients. Used independently or with assistance, it can reduce symptoms of respiratory insufficiency. Easy portability of manual resuscitation bags allows patients to use breath stacking to reduce dyspnea while away from home. Patients with severe bulbar symptoms are not able to use breath stacking because of poor glottic function and an inability to hold air in the chest between inhalations.

Glossopharyngeal Breathing

Glossopharyngeal breathing (GPB) is the "gulping" of boluses of air into the lungs. GPB, also known as "frog breathing," has the potential to increase lung volumes in ALS patients with respiratory insufficiency. GPB is accomplished by using the lips, tongue, and pharyngeal muscles to propel air past the glottis (Bach, 1994; Dail & Affeldt, 1955). Intact bulbar muscles are necessary for GPB as the tongue, soft palate, pharynx, and larynx are involved in the technique and the glottis must close after each gulp so air can be held in the lungs during subsequent breaths.

GPB assists spontaneous breathing in respiratory compromised ALS patients. It can be used for periods off noninvasive ventilation and is another tool that allows for breathing independence as the disease progresses. GPB has been studied in patients with postpolio respiratory insufficiency and DMD (Bach et al., 1987; Baydur et al., 1990). Each gulp ranges from 60 to 100 mL each, and six to nine gulps constitute one tidal volume breath (Bach, 2002a). Peak cough flow (PCF) and maximum inspiratory capacity have been increased in patients with spinal cord injury using GPB (Bianchi et al., 2004; Warren, 2002).

Abdominal Pressure Ventilator

The abdominal pressure ventilator, marketed as the Pneumobelt by Respironics (Murrysville, PA), can augment tidal volumes from 300 mL to as high as 1200 mL in spontaneously breathing patients (Bach & Alba, 1991). It has been used successfully in patients with DMD and anecdotal reports in patients with ALS are positive. It is less effective in patients with scoliosis and obesity (Bach, 2002b). For patients that require intermittent noninvasive ventilation during the day and who cannot or do not want to use NPPV with mask or nasal cushion interface, abdominal pressure ventilation is an option. Patients may find breathing feels more natural than with positive pressure chest expansion. Inhalation happens passively as thoracic pressure changes from ambient to negative with downward movement of the diaphragm.

To achieve a simulated breath, a cloth corset containing an inflatable rubber bladder is worn around the patient's abdomen. Tubing connects the rubber bladder to a positive pressure ventilator that inflates it intermittently. On the inspiratory cycle, air from the ventilator inflates the bladder, displacing the abdominal contents towards the diaphragm. (Inspiratory pressures of 15 to 45 cm H_2OH_2O are common.) On the exhalation cycle, the bladder deflates, allowing the abdomen and the diaphragm to move downward by gravity. Lung expansion occurs passively as air moves from the upper airway to the lower.

In order for abdominal pressure ventilation to work, the patient must sit at a $\geq$ 30- to 90-degree angle and must not lie flat. Active glossopharyngeal breathing can be combined with passive downward movement of diaphragm and abdomen to increase tidal volumes. The same mechanical ventilator used for volume expansion during the day can be used with a mask for respiratory assistance at night.

Mouthpiece Ventilation

Open-circuit mouthpiece ventilation (MPV) straddles the line between intermittent lung volume recruitment and intermittent noninvasive ventilation. Also referred to as mouthpiece intermittent positive pressure ventilation and more popularly as "sip ventilation," or "sip and puff ventilation," it provides portable daytime ventilatory support. MPV can be used for breath stacking to hyperinflate the lungs, increase vital capacity, improve expiratory flow rates to assist cough, and improve oxygenation (Kang & Bach, 2000). It is an alternative to tracheostomy and mechanical ventilation in patients with advanced neuromuscular disease and increasing need for respiratory assistance (Bach, 1993). Patients must have sufficient lip and oral-pharyngeal muscle strength to initiate a breath and maintain a seal while receiving a breath.

ALS patients with chronic respiratory insufficiency, for whom nocturnal NPPV is no longer sufficient, may find MPV an effective means of continuous noninvasive diurnal ventilation. The popularity of MPV is its portability (units are easily mounted on an electric wheelchair) and flexibility (ability to obtain as much ventilatory support as needed) (Boitano & Benditt, 2005). In addition, patients prefer its convenience, improved speech capability, comfort, and appearance to tracheostomy (Bach et al, 1993).

Method

MPV is accomplished using a single-limbed portable volume-cycled, pressure-triggered ventilator designed for home care use and an angled mouthpiece supported by a flexible support arm. Volume ventilators are open circuit systems with low-pressure alarms set to announce drop in pressure denoting significant leaks or tubing disconnection. The combination of an angled restriction or small bore tubing and sufficient inspiratory flow will generate enough system back pressure to defeat low-pressure alarms. (A 15-mm angled mouthpiece or foreshortened endotracheal tube can be used.) Coordinating the breath rate in assist/control mode with the patient's spontaneous respiratory rate eliminates the apnea alarm (Boitano & Benditt, 2005). The patient triggers the ventilator to inspiration by taking a "sip" from the mouthpiece positioned near the face. As leaks around the mouthpiece are common, tidal volumes are set higher than for closed-system invasive ventilation, generally in the 700- to 1200-mL range (Benditt, 2006b).

A detailed description of MPV can be found on the University of Washington website: http://www.uwtv.org/programs/displayevent.aspx?rID=4123&fID=853.

Bilevel Pressure Generators Versus Volume-Cycled Ventilators

MPV can be accomplished using NPPVs; however, the NPPV requires preset IPAP and EPAP settings resulting in variable tidal volumes. Deteriorating lung compliance common to neuromuscular disease progression results in decreased tidal volumes and the risk of underventilation. NPPV does not allow for varying patient tidal volumes needs during the day and cannot accommodate breath-stacking maneuvers. Maximum inspiratory pressures on most NPPV units vary from 25 to 35 cm H_2O and may be insufficient.

Volume ventilators can accommodate the higher pressures needed as muscles of inspiration continue to weaken. Volume ventilators also allow for a range of sensitivity adjustments for cycling to inspiration, thereby reducing the work required to access a machine breath. They can be used without positive end expiratory pressure if that option causes fatigue or discomfort in patients with ALS. In addition, the exhalation valve on volume ventilators reduces of chances of rebreathing exhaled CO_2.

MPV Procedure

Boitano and Benditt (2005) compared eight volume-cycled, pressure-triggered ventilators designed for home use to see which ones would best support MPV and what peak inspiratory flow rates would create enough system pressure to prevent low-pressure alarming. Six of eight ventilators commercially available in the United States were capable of accommodating open-circuit ventilation. For each ventilator, peak inspiratory flow (in liters per minute) or inspiratory time (I_t, in seconds) to prevent low-pressure alarming was determined at set tidal volumes (V_T) from 500 to 1000 mL. Based on the manufacturers' preset apnea duration, the minimum breaths per minute in A/C mode were determined to prevent alarm activation. The lower the set V_T the higher was the flow rate, and the lower the set V_T the lower was the I_t needed to maintain an open system without alarm activation. For the six portable volume ventilators capable of providing MPV, minimum breaths per minute ranged from one to six, with the lowest apnea duration (10 seconds) requiring the highest A/C rate (6 breaths per minute).

Clinicians have a range of portable ventilators to choose from when recommending MPV to patients. Other considerations are weight, dimensions (for use on wheelchair), internal battery, and duration of internal battery life.

Sample settings for MPV with volume-cycled, pressure-triggered ventilator are the following:

Mode: Assist Control (A/C)
Rate: 4 to 5 breaths
V_T: 500 mL (titrate for patient comfort)
Low airway pressure alarm: minimum setting (2 to 3 cm H_2O)
High airway pressure alarm: maximum
Sensitivity: to allow patient to easily access a breath by sipping on the mouthpiece

---

AIRWAY SECRETION MANAGEMENT

Patients with ALS who have developed weak expiratory and abdominal muscles in addition to weak inspiratory muscles will have difficulty coughing and clearing the airway of retained secretions. This can be seen clinically by observing the outward movement of the abdomen during coughing and objectively measured by PCF or peak expiratory pressure. Healthy individuals can produce a PCF as high as 720 liters per minute (LPM) (Homnick, 2007). A PCF of at least 270 LPM is necessary to manage increased secretions during upper respiratory tract infection in patients with DMD (Bach & Saporito, 1996). A minimum PCF of 160 LPM is necessary for weaning patients from mechanical ventilation (Bach et al., 1997).

In 2006, the American College of Chest Physicians published clinical practice guidelines for airway clearance therapies (McCool & Rosen, 2006). Three of the 10 recommendations were for patients with neuromuscular disease or expiratory muscle weakness: expiratory muscle strength training, manual cough assist, and mechanical cough assist. Evidence for these recommendations were based largely on expert opinion or observational studies, lacked randomized controlled trials, and were underpowered statistically (McCrory & Rosen, 2006). Expiratory muscle strength training and manual cough assist showed only a small benefit, whereas mechanical cough assist showed clear benefit but with the risk of harm. The remainder of this chapter covers secretion mobilization and cough assistive therapies currently in use in the United States.

Mechanically Assisted Cough

Mechanical insufflation-exsufflation (MI-E) has been used for secretion management in rudimentary forms for over 60 years. The prototype of the Cough Assist (Respironics, Murraysville, PA) used today was the Cof-flator, first marketed by Original Equipment Manufacturing, known as the OEM Company (Norwalk, CT), in 1953 and used predominantly with poliomyelitis patients. After falling out of clinical favor, it was redesigned and marketed by J.H. Emerson (Cambridge, MA) as the Cough Assist In-Exsufflator in 1993 (Bach, 2002). With a growing trend toward noninvasive ventilation and away from tracheostomy and mechanical ventilation, MI-E use for secretion mobilization is on the rise. There are no accepted guidelines for when to initiate MI-E, but a protocol instituted by Bach et al. (1997) recommends use when PCFs are <270 LPM.

MI-E assists people with weakened respiratory muscles and ineffective cough clear retained bronchopulmonary secretions by gradually applying positive pressure to the airway, inflating the lungs, and then rapidly shifting to negative pressure, removing the insufflated volume. The rapid shift in pressure produces a high expiratory flow rate, much like a cough. Each cough cycle consists of an insufflation phase, an exsufflation phase, and a pause phase. Current models can be operated either manually or in automatic mode by using preset insufflation, exsufflation, and pause cycle times. High and low insufflation flow settings are an option.

The Cough Assist is an electrically powered device. MI-E can be used with an air-cushioned face mask, mouth piece, or tracheostomy tube with cuff inflated. Smooth bore tubing allows pressurized air to flow between the unit and patient. Settings are independent of one another and offer a range of options. These include the following: insufflation and exsufflation pressure, insufflation and exsufflation time (in seconds), pause time, and high or low flow.

Pressures of +40/−40 cm H_2O are recommended by the manufacturer for effective secretion removal, although pressures of +60/−60 cm H_2O may be required as lung compliance decreases. Exsufflation time is generally set at half the insufflation time. At the lower flow setting, a 3- to

4-second insufflation time is recommended. Total cycle time should not exceed 7 seconds (Haas et al., 2007). Manually assisted cough (abdominal thrust) may be applied during the exsufflation cycle to augment expiratory flow.

Haas et al. (2007) reviewed 10 studies (published between 1993 and 2006) that compared MI-E with other methods of secretion mobilization. Six of these studies included patients with ALS, and two of these six compared ALS patients with and without bulbar dysfunction. Only one study was a randomized crossover trial—the level of evidence was low, and the research conclusions were not unanimous; however, in their summary, Haas et al. concluded that MI-E appears to be well tolerated and safe. PCFs, the major outcome measure in each study, are as fast or faster than those achieved with manually assisted cough, and inspired volumes rivaled breath stacking and GPB techniques. Upper-airway collapse on exsufflation with advanced bulbar muscle weakness or lack of patient cooperation appeared to be the only obstacles to using MI-E.

MI-E treatment recommendations for ALS patients are as follows:

- Five to six breaths = one cycle
- Five to six cycles = one treatment
- Cough (independently or with manual assistance) to swallow or expectorate secretions
- Rest for 30 to 45 seconds between cycles at a normal respiratory rate
- Perform three treatments each day

Frequency recommendations for patients with pneumonia or acute respiratory infection with mucus production are as follows:

- One treatment in the morning while lying in bed (to assist in mobilizing secretions that have pooled in the airway during the night)
- One treatment an hour before going to bed (to clear the lungs prior to sleep)
- Treatments during the day as needed to promote secretion clearance and prevent pulmonary congestion

---

Because lack of familiarity with MI-E can be a barrier to use, it is recommended that patients and family members practice using the device so that they will be comfortable with it and be able to use it when it is needed for lung expansion and secretion removal.

HIGH-FREQUENCY CHEST WALL COMPRESSION

High-frequency chest wall compression (HFCWC) is an airway clearance technique that uses small, rapid compressions to produce mini coughs. HFCWC is frequently referred to as high-frequency chest wall oscillation and is abbreviated HFCWO. Chatburn (2007) pointed out that true chest wall oscillation is provided solely by the Hayek oscillator system (Medivent International, London, UK), which uses a rigid chest cuirass (shell) to deliver biphasic compressions to the chest wall, augmenting both inspiration and exhalation, at frequencies of 1 to 17 Hz.

The Vest (Hill Rom, St. Paul, MN) Airway Clearance System generates high-frequency chest wall compressions at pressures from 5 to 20 cm H_2O and oscillations between 2 to 25 Hz to generate airway flows up to 1.6 L/sec. A cloth vest fastened snugly around the patient's chest is connected to an air pulse generator by two tubes. By rapidly compressing and releasing the chest wall (up to 25 times per second), HFCWC dislodges mucus from the airway. The Vest compresses the chest from functional residual capacity to below initial lung volume, allowing chest wall recoil to bring the lungs back to resting volume. This is the system currently used in research in muscular dystrophy and ALS to study airway clearance through external chest wall compression.

According to the Hill Rom (St. Paul, MN) product literature, oscillating airflow in the lower airway augments the natural function of the mucociliary escalator and reduces the viscosity of mucus. Through rapid compressions The Vest generates increased airflow velocities that create cough-like shear force and decreases secretion viscosity (Haas et al., 2007). Together, volume, flow, and frequency combine to move mucus secretions from the smaller to the larger airways where they can be swallowed or expectorated. Recommended treatment times are 20 to 30 minutes at different compression frequencies with pauses for assisted coughing (Chatburn, 2007).

The majority of randomized controlled trials and long-term nonrandomized trials comparing HFCWC to chest physical therapy (CPT) have been conducted in cystic fibrosis (CF) and pediatric patients (Scherer et al., 1998; Stites et al., 2006). These studies found HFCWC to be as effective as and possibly better than standard CPT. Three studies have been conducted in patients with ALS. Chaisson et al. (2006) found no significant difference in the rate of FVC decline in patients who received twice daily HFCWC and those receiving standard therapy. Lange et al. (2006) found HFCWC users had less breathlessness and coughed more at night than those who received standard therapy. In a subgroup of patients with a baseline FVC of 40% to 70% of predicted, HFCWC users had a slower decline in FVC and capnography results than those with FVC greater than 70%. Jackson et al. (2006) also reported increased patient comfort but no studies have shown improvement in FVC or rate of decline in FVC over time. HFCWC appeared safe and was well tolerated. At this time, there are no published clinical data to support the use of HFCWC as a maintenance therapy for secretion clearance in ALS. HFCWC is not a substitute for an effective cough and therefore may be hazardous if mobilized secretions cannot be expectorated because of severe neuromuscular dysfunction (Rubin, 2007).

Intrapulmonary Percussive Ventilation

The intrapulmonary percussive ventilator (IPV) is a low-frequency air-column oscillator that delivers high-flow minibursts of air while providing aerosolized medication to the airways. The IPV is able to vibrate the airways internally by generating flow rates of 100 to 300 cycles per minute (1.7 to 5 Hz) while the patient breaths spontaneously through a mouthpiece. IPV is used to mobilize and clear retained secretions and treat patchy atelectasis (Haas et al., 2007). Treatments generally last 15 to 20 minutes.

IPV was invented by Dr. Forrest Bird to deliver aerosolized bronchodilators to patients with chronic obstructive pulmonary disease. It was first described in *Respiratory Care*, journal of the American Association for Respiratory Care in 1985 (McInturff et al.). The current version of IPV is marketed as the Percussionator and is sold by the Percussionaire Corporation (Sagle, ID).

Studies with IPV have been conducted in CF and DMD. Varekojis et al. (2003) found IPV compared favorably with CPT and HFCWC in patients with CF, whereas Marks et al. (2004) found no statistically significant difference in IPV and standard CPT in this patient population. Toussaint et al. (2003) conducted a randomized crossover trial with DMD patients that compared assisted mucus clearance technique with and without IPV. Their results showed mean mucus production (based on weight of mucus expectorated) to be significantly higher with IPV use. One randomized controlled trial in pediatric patients with neuromuscular disease comparing prophylactic IPV with incentive spirometry showed less antibiotic use, shorter hospitalization days, and fewer missed school days with IPV. IPV was safe and well tolerated by the patients in this study (Reardon et al., 2005). No studies of IPV in ALS have been published.

A single-patient use, disposable IPV unit, PercussiveNeb (Vortran Medical Technology, Sacramento, CA) is also available for home use. It is powered by a high-flow air compressor and produces frequencies of 11 to 30 Hz. It is also designed to mobilize secretions while delivering aerosolized medication.

All mucus clearance devices are considered investigational in ALS because scientific data showing health benefits in this patient population are lacking. The published medical literature consists of small, randomized studies with crossover designs of short duration. To date, there are no long-term studies that show improvement in lung function or decrease in pulmonary exacerbations that led to hospitalization. For these reasons, some insurance companies may not be willing to reimburse durable medical equipment companies for mucus clearance devices in the home.

COUGH TECHNIQUES

The mechanisms and function of cough and the physiology of airway mucus are detailed in Chapter 6. In this chapter, we have been concerned with techniques for expanding the lungs and mobilizing troublesome secretions. Successful expectoration of mucus depends on several factors: expiratory flow rates, volume of airway secretions, accumulation (pooling), mucus viscosity, and site of production. In this final section, we explore assisted and independent cough techniques that can be used to augment the therapies described previously.

Manual Cough Assist

Manual cough assist refers to the manual application of pressure to the upper abdomen or lower thorax at end inspiration. This technique is also called "quad" coughing because it is used with quadriplegic patients who have suffered spinal cord injuries and are unable to generate an effective cough (Kirby et al., 1966). The goal is to mimic contraction of the abdominal muscles and push the diaphragm upward, displacing lung volume and increasing PCF. The technique is similar to the abdominal thrust performed when a choking victim has lost consciousness and is supine.

Technique and timing are essential for effective manual cough assist. The patient should be sitting at approximately 45 degrees. Facing the patient, the caregiver places both hands over the epigastric area. The patient inhales to maximum capacity and at end-inspiration the caregiver pushes diagonally upward in a quick, yet smooth, motion as the patient coughs. Patients and caregivers can coordinate for best effect. Caregiver verbal coaching will aid in coordinating inspiration and cough on exhalation.

Manual cough assist is used as an adjunct to the volume expansion techniques described at the beginning of the chapter. Two studies in ALS using manual assisted cough with MI-E and breath stacking showed increased unassisted PCFs (Mustfa et al., 2003; Sancho et al., 2004). These studies, too, were crossover and randomized crossover trials with small samples and short duration, and thus, it is unclear what the long-term benefits might be; however, it is another tool in a disease in which patient comfort, symptom management, and avoidance of acute exacerbations are the goals.

Patients with weakened bulbar muscles are at risk for choking. Instructing patients and caregivers in manual cough assist technique early in the disease course will allow them to practice and be ready to use it in an emergency as well as for routine secretion management. Armed with only a manual resuscitation bag and proficiency in manual cough assist, caregivers will be able to provide the most basic, and perhaps the most effective, volume expansion and secretion mobilization techniques available.

Self Heimlich

ALS patients with weakened bulbar muscles at risk for choking who are able to stand should be instructed in methods to increase PCFs independently. Pressing the abdomen quickly into a chair back or other rigid surface will increase peak air flow and dislodge food or tenacious saliva from the back of the throat. Wearing and activating an emergency alarm pendant is an added safety precaution for those at risk of choking who are home alone.

Self-Seated Cough Assist

Patients can increase peak expiratory flow by using a pillow to compress the abdomen during exhalation. Patients should sit in a chair with feet firmly on the floor or on a stool. A pillow is placed over the abdomen and is supported by both arms. The patient inhales to maximum capacity and exhales while bending over and tightly hugging the pillow. This should be repeated five to six times. This sequence is followed by a coughing maneuver while bending over and compressing the abdomen with the pillow, and it is repeated two to three times. The self-sitting cough maneuver can follow breath stacking. Patients able to self-administer volume expansion, secretion mobilization, and coughing techniques may gain confidence in their abilities to manage their airways and prevent potential respiratory infection.

Forced Exhalation Techniques

During forced expiration, pressure surrounding the airway is higher than pressure within the airway. The transmural pressure results in airway narrowing and increased airflow velocity. This creates a high shear rate that varies inversely with mucus transport because of increased mucus viscosity (van der Schans, 2007). It is hypothesized then that brief, repetitive coughs (two to three) will be more effective than coughs with longer duration because of reduced mucus viscosity and better mucus transport.

Assisted forced exhalation can be accomplished with the patient using a closed glottis (cough) or open glottis (huff). Effective cough and huff require a strong contraction of the expiratory muscles or in their absence a fast and forceful abdominal thrust coordinated with glottic opening or vocalizing of the word "huff." Cough or huff can begin at low, middle, or high lung volumes (van der Schans, 2007). Coordination is key and may be more easily accomplished with the huff technique.

Active Cycle Breathing Technique

The active cycle breathing technique (ACBT) combines relaxed diaphragmatic breathing, lung expansion, and forced expiratory technique (huff from middle to low lung volumes). ACBT has been used in conjunction with postural drainage in patients with CF (Fink, 2007). It is designed to improve pulmonary function and airway clearance and compares favorably with CPT, positive expiratory pressure, and oscillating positive expiratory pressure (Flutter or Acapella) in effectiveness.

ACBT was designed for spontaneously breathing patients and may be adopted for those with ALS. Patients and caregivers can combine breath stacking maneuvers and forced expiratory techniques with abdominal thrusts. ACBT could be recommended early in the disease process, for example, when FVC falls to 80% of predicted, when the patient can perform it independently. As ALS progresses, patients and caregivers can work together for volume expansion and secretion clearance. ACBT can be used for prophylaxis to prevent infection caused by atelectasis but may be used for secretion mobilization if respiratory tract infection occurs.

The procedure for active cycle of breathing with diaphragmatic muscle weakness is as follows:

1. Put the patient in a relaxed sitting or reclining position.
2. Have several minutes of relaxed breathing with diaphragm, if possible.
3. Provide three to four maximum inhalations with manual resuscitation bag (breath stacking) ending with 4-second breath hold. Allow passive, relaxed exhalations.
4. Use relaxed breathing,
5. Repeat three to four maximum inhalations with resuscitation bag, breath hold, passive exhalation.
6. Use relaxed breathing,
7. Perform two to three huffs with abdominal thrust starting at a lower volume, followed by two to three huffs with abdominal thrust at a higher volume.
8. Return to relaxed breathing.
9. Repeat sequence two to four times, as tolerated.

Adapted from Fink (2007).

NEW THERAPIES

Diaphragmatic Pacing System

A multicenter clinical trial is underway to determine the effectiveness of reducing the loss of vital capacity in ALS through therapeutic electro-stimulation of the diaphragm and phrenic nerves. In the diaphragmatic pacing system (DPS), four electrodes are placed on the diaphragm using minimally invasive laparoscopic technique. The diaphragm is conditioned through electrostimulation, which increases diaphragm muscle thickness. Initial results showed greater diaphragm excursion with diaphragm stimu-lation than under maximal voluntary effort by study participants. Improve-ment in posterior lobe lung ventilation, increase in lung compliance, and decreased work of breathing were also noted with DPS (Onders et al., 2007).

The goal of therapeutic DPS is to prolong life in ALS through the preservation of muscle mass and delay of respiratory failure. Preliminary results showed an average rate of decline of FVC of 1.3% per month from preimplantation decline of 3.1% a month (Onders et al., 2007). Researchers hope to improve nocturnal ventilation in patients with ALS through the use of DPS.

SUMMARY

Joshua Benditt of University of Washington, Seattle, pays a high compli-ment to RCPs when he recommends care of the neuromuscular patient by a healthcare team lead by a respiratory therapist (Benditt, 2006b). When managing the ventilation needs of patients with ALS, a detailed knowledge of microprocessor ventilators and the ability to adapt them creatively to noninvasive use is but one example. Patients with ALS need a variety of techniques and devices for volume expansion and airway clearance that range from simple to complex. Recommendations for respiratory and cough assistance must be tailored to the individual patient—their abilities, lung function status, personality, and their desired outcome. Flexibility and adaptability are key. RCPs are known for "high tech and high touch," meaning that they bring state-of-the-art technology in respiratory care, compassion, and healing together for the benefit of patients.

There are no definitive studies of mucus clearance devices in ALS. Results of the published short-term studies are largely inconclusive. Because most studies have been conducted on patients with chronic obstructive pulmonary disease, CF, and DMD, health benefits to patients with ALS must be inferred. There is a great deal of heterogeneity among these diseases and within the diseases themselves that make comparisons difficult.

Hess (2007) reminds RCPs that a lack of evidence does not necessarily mean lack of benefit. He poses basic questions that clinicians should ask themselves before recommending secretion clearance therapy and for evaluating its benefit. In order of priority, they are paraphrased here:

- What is the pathophysiological basis for recommending secretion mobilization therapy?
- Are airway secretions affecting lung function or gas exchange in any meaningful way?
- Are there potential adverse effects from therapy?
- What therapy technique is likely to provide the greatest benefit?
- Is the cost of therapy going to be covered by third-party insurers?
- What is the patient preference for one therapy over another or for any therapy at all?

REFERENCES

Bach JR. A comparison of long-term ventilatory support alternatives from the perspective of patient and caregiver. *Chest* 1993;104:1702–1706.

Bach JR. Update and perspectives on noninvasive respiratory muscle aids: I: the inspiratory aids. *Chest* 1994;105:1230–1240.

Bach JR. Noninvasive respiratory muscle aids and intervention goals. In Bach J (ed.). *Noninvasive Mechanical Ventilation.* Philadelphia: Hanley and Belfus; 2002a, pp. 129–163.

Bach JR. The history of mechanical ventilation and respiratory muscle aids. In Bach JR (ed.). *Noninvasive Mechanical Ventilation.* Philadelphia: Hanley and Belfus; 2002b, pp. 45–72.

Bach JR, Alba AS. Total ventilatory support by intermittent abdominal pressure ventilator. *Chest* 1991;99:630–636.

Bach JR, Saporito LR. Criteria for extubation and tracheostomy tube removal for patients with ventilatory failure: a different approach to weaning. *Chest* 1996;110: 1566–1571.

Bach J, Alba AS, Brodofsky E, et al. Glossopharyngeal breathing and non-invasive aids in the management of post-polio respiratory insufficiency. *Birth Defects* 1987;23:99–113.

Bach JR, Alba AS, Saporito LR. Intermittent positive pressure ventilation via mouth as an alternative to tracheostomy for 257 ventilator patients. *Chest* 1993;103: 174–182.

Bach JR, Ishikawa U, Kim H. Prevention of pulmonary morbidity for patients with Duchenne muscular dystrophy. *Chest* 1997;112:1024–1028.

Baydur A, Gilgoff I, Prentice W, et al. Decline in respiratory function and experience with long-term assisted ventilation in advanced Duchenne's muscular dystrophy. *Chest* 1990;98:884–889.

Benditt JO. The neuromuscular respiratory system: physiology, pathophysiology, and a respiratory care approach to patients. *Respir Care* 2006a;51:829–839.

Benditt JO. Full-time noninvasive ventilation: possible and desirable. *Respir Care* 2006b;51:1012–1015.

Bianchi C, Grandi M, Felisari G. Efficacy of glossopharyngeal breathing for a ventilator-dependent, high-level tetraplegic patient after cervical cord trauma resection and tracheostomy. *Am J Phys Med Rehabil* 2004;83:216–219.

Boitano LJ, Benditt JO. An evaluation of home volume ventilators that support open-circuit mouthpiece ventilation. *Respir Care* 2005;50:1457–1461.

Chaisson KM, Walsh S, Simmons Z, Vender RL. A clinical pilot study: high frequency chest wall oscillation airway clearance in patients with amyotrophic lateral sclerosis. *Amyotrophic Lateral Sclerosis* 2006;7:107–111.

Chatburn RL. High-frequency assisted airway clearance. *Respir Care* 2007;52:1224–1235.

Dail CW, Affeldt JE. Clinical aspects of glossopharyngeal breathing. *JAMA* 1955; 158(6):445–449.

Fink JB. Forced expiratory technique, directed cough, and autogenic drainage. *Respir Care* 2007;52:1210–1221.

Haas CF, Loik PS, Gay SE. Airway clearance applications in the elderly and in patients with neurologic and neuromuscular compromise. *Respir Care* 2007;52: 1362–1381.

Hess DR. Secretion clearance techniques: absence of proof or proof of absence? *Respir Care* 2002;47:757–758.

Hess DR. Airway clearance: physiology, pharmacology, techniques, and practice (conference summary). *Respir Care* 2007;52:1392–1396.

Homnick DN. Mechanical insufflation-exsufflation for airway mucus clearance. *Respir Care* 2007;52(10):1296–1305.

Jackson CE, Moore DH, Kittrell P, Ensrud E. High frequency chest wall oscillation therapy in amyotrophic lateral sclerosis. *J Clin Neuromusc Dis* 2006;8:60–64.

Kang SW, Bach JR. Maximum insufflation capacity. *Chest* 2000;118:61–65.

Kirby N, Barnerias MS, Siebeus AA. An evaluation of assisted cough in quadriparetic patients. *Arch Phys Med Rehabil* 1966:705–710.

Lange DJ, Lechtzin N, Davey C, et al. High-frequency chest wall oscillation airway clearance in patients with ALS: an exploratory randomized, controlled trial. *Neurology* 2006;67:991–997.

Lechtzin N, Shade D, Clawson L, et al. Supramaximal inflation improves lung compliance in subjects with amyotrophic lateral sclerosis. *Chest* 2006;129:1322–1329.

Marks JH, Hare KL, Saunders RA, et al. Pulmonary function and sputum production in patients with cystic fibrosis: a pilot study comparing the Percussive Tech HF device and stand chest physiotherapy. *Chest* 2004;125:1507–1511.

McCool FD, Rosen MJ. Nonpharmacologic airway clearance therapies: ACCP evidence-based clinical practice guidelines. *Chest* 2006;129(1 Suppl):250S–259S.

McCrory FD, Rosen MJ. Methodology and grading of the evidence for the diagnosis and management of cough: ACCP evidence-based clinical practice guidelines. *Chest* 2006;129(1 Suppl):28S–32S.

McInturff SL, Shaw LI, Hodgkin JE, et al. Intrapulmonary percussive ventilation (IPV) in the treatment of COPD. *Respir Care* 1985;30:885.

Mustfa N, Aiello M, Lyall RA, et al. Cough augmentation in amyotrophic lateral sclerosis. *Neurology* 2003;61:1285–1287.

Onders R, Schilz R, Katirji B, et al. Improvement of respiratory muscle deterioration using the diaphragm pacing stimulation (DPS) system in patients with amyotrophic lateral sclerosis (ALS) (abstract). *Chest* 2007;132:575.

Reardon CC, Christiansen D, Barnett ED, et al. Intrapulmonary percussion ventilation vs incentive spirometry for children with neuromuscular disease. *Arch Pediatr Adolesc Med* 2005;159:526–531.

Rubin BK. High frequency external chest wall compression for secretion clearance: shake it. But don't break it. *Respir Care* 2007;52:982–983.

Sancho J, Severa E, Diaz J, Marin J. Efficacy of mechanical insufflation-exsufflation in medically stable patients with amyotrophic lateral sclerosis. *Chest* 2004;125:1400–1405.

Scherer TA, Barandum J, Martinez E, et al. Effect of high-frequency oral airway and chest wall oscillation and conventional chest physical therapy on expectoration in patients with stable cystic fibrosis. *Chest* 1998;113:1019–1027.

Stites SW, Perry GV, Peddicord T, et al. Effect of high-frequency chest wall oscillation on the ventral and peripheral distribution of aerosolized diethylene thiamine penta-acetic acid as compared to stand chest physiotherapy in cystic fibrosis. *Chest* 2006;129:712–717.

Toussaint M, De Win H, Steens M, et al. Effect of intrapulmonary percussive ventilation on mucous clearance in Duchenne muscular dystrophy patients: a preliminary report. *Respir Care* 2003;48:940–947.

Toussaint M, Steens M, Wasteels G, Soudon P. Diurnal ventilation via mouthpiece: survival in end-stage Duchenne patients. *Eur Respir J* 2006;28:549–555.

Trebbia G, Lacombe M, Fermanian C, et al. Cough determinants in patients with neuromuscular disease. *Respir Physiol Neurobiol* 2005;146:291–300.

van der Schans CP. Bronchial mucous transport. *Respir Care* 2007;52:1150–1156.

Varekojis SM, Douce FH, Flucke RL, et al. A comparison of the therapeutic effectiveness of and preference for postural drainage and percussion, intrapulmonary percussive ventilation, and high-frequency chest wall compression in hospitalized cystic fibrosis patients. *Respir Care* 2003;48:24–28.

Warren VC. Glossopharyngeal and neck accessory muscle breathing in a young adult with C2 complete tetraplegia resulting in ventilator dependency. *Phys Ther* 2002;82:590–600.

QUESTIONS FOR RESEARCH

1. What are the risks of mobilizing secretions in patients with ALS or other neuromuscular diseases who have impaired ability to cough?

2. Sputum weight is used as a proxy for health outcomes when studying mucus clearance devices. How reliable and valid is this as an outcome measure? What other end point could be used to evaluate the effectiveness of mucus clearance therapies?

3. Quality of life is a measurement requirement for Food and Drug Administration approval of respiratory therapies. How is quality of life measured in ALS? What combination of questionnaires and scales could be used to quantify patient-reported symptoms?

CHAPTER 8

Noninvasive Positive Pressure Ventilation

CHAPTER OUTLINE

INTRODUCTION

Volume expansion and alveolar recruitment strategies have been covered in Chapter 7, but noninvasive positive pressure ventilation (NPPV) deserves a chapter of its own. Of the symptom management strategies currently available for amyotrophic lateral sclerosis (ALS), noninvasive ventilation for treatment of respiratory insufficiency and percutaneous endoscopic gastrostomy (PEG) for nutrition maintenance are the two that show promise in not only improving quality of life (QoL) but also increasing life expectancy (Bourke et al., 2006; Mazzini et al., 1995).

HISTORY

French researcher Rideau and colleagues (1981) pioneered the management of respiratory insufficiency by means of noninvasive mask ventilation. In the United States, Bach et al. (1987) published articles on its benefits and have continued to champion its use (Bach, 2002). The majority of research on noninvasive positive pressure ventilation (NPPV) in neuromuscular disease has been done with Duchenne muscular dystrophy. In this population, NPPV has been shown to impact survival time positively (Simonds et al., 1998).

Noninvasive ventilation via a mask has been proposed for the treatment of acute respiratory failure since the late 1980s (Meduri et al., 1989). Increasing acceptance of NPPV in the management of acute respiratory failure in chronic obstructive pulmonary disease (COPD) has reduced the cost and complications of endotracheal intubation (Kaplan, 1991 Rubenfeld, 1997). Its success in treating post-extubation respiratory insufficiency and weaning from mechanical ventilation has also been documented (Nava et al., 1998; Udwadia et al., 1992). Congruent with the emergence of NPPV as a treatment modality, *Respiratory Care*, the journal of the American Association for Respiratory Care, hosted a consensus conference in 1997 to explore its uses and benefits. Since that time, respiratory assistive devices have continued to evolve. Pressure-targeted devices allow clinicians to adjust inspiratory time and rise time, as well as maximum inspiratory positive airway pressure (IPAP) and expiratory positive airway pressure (EPAP) and timed breaths for optimal support. Improved pressure-flow characteristics, leak compensation, and ease of moving from end inspiration to exhalation have improved patient comfort and control. Bilevel pressure ventilators are effective in treating patients with chronic respiratory insufficiency and are comparable to critical care ventilators (Vitacca, 2002).

NPPV units for home use have become smaller and lighter in weight and have integrated heated humidifiers. They can be adapted to battery power and mounted on motorized wheelchairs. These modifications allow people with ALS to be highly mobile while they receive intermittent or continuous ventilatory support. For people who do not desire tracheostomy, it is an option that can reduce signs and symptoms of chronic respiratory insufficiency. In ALS, the use of NPPV is palliative and is currently used primarily to improve QoL, not prolong it; however, a recent retrospective cohort study (Lechtzin et al., 2007) and a randomized, controlled trial (Bourke et al., 2006) have shown survival benefits, especially with early intervention.

DEFINITION

One can find interchangeable terms for noninvasive ventilation in the medical literature: noninvasive bilevel pressure ventilation; noninvasive positive pressure ventilation, abbreviated NIPPV or NPPV; noninvasive ventilation; and pressure support ventilation (PSV). These terms and acronyms refer not to the device itself but the mode of ventilation. BiPAP, an abbreviation for bilevel positive airway pressure, is a registered trademark of Respironics, Inc., now part of the Philips Company.

NPPV is a form of PSV. Inspiratory flow delivers a volume greater than patients with respiratory muscle weakness can achieve without assistance. Expiratory flow is set lower than inspiratory level, allowing for ease of exhalation while maintaining continuous thoracic pressure and alveolar recruitment. Pressure support is the difference between the set pressure levels. What is common to all of the previous terminology is *ventilation*. All patients with progressive neuromuscular disease, even those able to breathe spontaneously, need back up ventilation. Using the spontaneous/timed (S/T) option assures that patients will receive adequate minute ventilation if they become apneic or are unable to trigger inspiration due to diaphragmatic muscle weakness, especially during deep, restorative levels of sleep.

PHYSIOLOGICAL EFFECTS OF NPPV

NPPV decreases the work required to maintain adequate ventilation. Significant weight loss, increased respiratory rate and heart rate, and increased fatigue are all surrogate markers of increased work of breathing.

Volume Expansion

In spontaneously breathing patients, NPPV is used to augment lung volumes lost through pulmonary compromise. A loss of respiratory muscle innervation leads to reduced vital capacity and resting tidal volumes. Patients respond by increasing their respiratory rate to achieve appropriate minute ventilation. They may experience inadequate ventilation as dyspnea at rest or with exercise, orthopnea, agitation, anxiety, and loss of a sense of well-being. Depression and changes in cognitive function have been noted in patients with respiratory insufficiency (Newsom-Davis et al., 2001). Oxygen desaturation results in tachycardia and increased cardiac workload.

Alveolar Recruitment

NPPV improves gas exchange and symptoms of respiratory insufficiency by improving alveolar ventilation. Positive inspiratory pressure increases mean airway pressure, improving oxygenation by recruiting underinflated lung units. The lower level of expiratory pressure assures that recruited lung units are maintained while allowing ease of exhalation. Reduced cardiac oxygen demand allows improved oxygen delivery to muscle and tissue sites.

Nocturnal NPPV Use and Improved Diurnal Improvement

The mechanisms by which nocturnal NPPV improves daytime functioning in ALS are speculative. Three of the most widely held hypotheses are briefly summarized here:

- Patients with ALS have reduced lung compliance, as evaluated by static expiratory lung measures. This suggests that atelectasis or increased alveolar surface tension is present in ALS patients with chronic diaphragmatic muscle weakness. This results in increased work of breathing (Lechtzin et al., 2006). Recruitment of underinflated alveoli allows for better distribution of gas exchange, improving oxygenation and elimination of carbon dioxide. This can be accomplished by increasing mean airway pressure with IPAP and maintaining a lower, consistent pressure with EPAP. Decreased dyspnea and improved sleep quality and daytime functioning often result.
- Nocturnal hypercapnia and hypoxemia lead to a blunting of central respiratory drive. This results in compensatory daytime hypoventilation and blunting of central chemoreceptor response to elevated $PaCO_2$. Nocturnal NPPV "resets" the central control mechanisms and reduces buffering bicarbonate so that daytime increases in $PaCO_2$ lead to appropriate increases in minute ventilation (Benditt, 2006).
- Nocturnal NPPV rests fatigued respiratory muscles and may improve daytime inspiratory muscle endurance. Measures of transdiaphragmatic pressure and pressure-time indices in acute exacerbation of COPD have shown NPPV to reduce inspiratory muscle activity (Brochard et al., 1990).

BENEFITS OF NPPV

NPPV may slow decline in vital capacity (Kleopa, 1999) and increase lung compliance (Lechtzin et al., 2006), thereby prolonging survival and reducing dyspnea. For these reasons, the American Academy of Neurology and American College of Chest Physicians recommend initiation of NPPV after forced vital capacity (FVC) drops below 50% of predicted values, MIP maximum inspiratory pressure falls below −60 cm H_2O or daytime $PaCO_2$ increases above 45 mm Hg, whichever comes first.

Survival

Patients able to tolerate NPPV have been shown to have a slower rate of decline in their FVC (Lo CoCo et al., 2006). NPPV use of more than 4 hours per day has been shown to increase survival by 7 months (Kleopa, 1999) and by a mean of 11 months when NPPV was initiated at the first sign of nocturnal oxygen desaturation (Pinto et al., 1995). The longest survival benefit reported in ALS with NPPV use is 20 months (Aboussouan et al., 2001).

Quality of Life (QoL)

Improvement in QoL for patients with ALS reflects improvement in symptomatic nocturnal hypoventilation, as measured by the Sleep Apnea QoL scale and Epworth sleepiness scale (Bourke et al., 2003; Lyall et al., 2001). Increased lung expansion decreases work of breathing and diurnal dyspnea. In addition, users of NPPV have reported improvements in vitality, energy, and general health (Bourke et al.).

Pulmonary Function

If used more than 4 hours per day, NPPV has been shown to slow the decline of pulmonary function measured by FVC (Kleopa, 1999); however, this conclusion has not been reached in other studies that compared pulmonary function decline in patients able to use NPPV successfully and those who were intolerant (Aboussouan et al.).

Sleep-Disordered Breathing

The diaphragm is the major muscle of respiration. In rapid eye movement (REM) sleep, it is the only respiratory muscle active. External intercostals, scalenes, and sternomastoids are inactive during this level of sleep. Progressive denervation of the diaphragm leads to decreased vital capacity and is more greatly pronounced in the supine position. Respiratory insufficiency at night caused by a weakened diaphragm and a loss of other inspiratory and accessory muscles leads to hypoxemia and hypercapnia.

In obstructive sleep apnea (OSA), partial or total blockage of the upper airway by the tongue, soft palate, or other oropharyngeal structures causes intermittent apneas and hypopneas. Hypoxemia and disruption of REM sleep result as the body is pulled from a deep, restorative level of sleep into a lighter one so that accessory muscle use can be activated and ventilation restored. Upper-airway obstruction is not a hallmark of neuromuscular disease, but OSA may be a preexisting condition; however, sleep-disordered breathing caused by denervation of upper-airway muscles, especially the tongue and soft palate, may be present. Fragmented sleep, poor sleep quality, and changes in sleep architecture caused by upper airway obstruction can be successfully treated with NPPV.

The most objective method of assessing nocturnal respiratory insufficiency and sleep quality is polysomnography. Neuromuscular patients may be referred to a sleep center for documentation of respiratory events and initiation of NPPV. ALS patients may find that participating in an overnight sleep study is difficult because of generalized weakness and decreased mobility. The wait time for appointments can be long, and if the patient does not have comprehensive health insurance, it will be expensive. Most sleep technologists are trained to titrate noninvasive positive pressures until respiratory events (apneas, hypopneas, desaturations) are eliminated. This may result in the use of continuous positive airway pressure (CPAP) or EPAP settings that are too high for the comfort of neuromuscular patients. Because ALS is progressive, NPPV pressures will need to be regularly assessed and adjusted, which entails return trips to the sleep laboratory.

For these reasons, more pulmonologists, neurologists, respiratory care practitioners (RCPs), and nurses are now documenting patient-reported symptoms of nocturnal hypoventilation during each clinic visit. For example, hypoxemia should be suspected if patients report morning headaches as cerebral vasodilatation occurs in response to low levels of oxygen. Relaxation of smooth muscle of the cerebral vasculature allows for increased blood flow and oxygen delivery to brain tissue, and the resulting pressure may create a headache. Morning headaches and orthopnea should prompt clinicians to obtain FVC and MIP values in the supine as well as upright positions, and NPPV should be discussed with the patient and family. These and other patient-reported symptoms are covered in detail in Chapter 5.

TIMING OF NPPV

The recommendation for NPPV is made once FVC drops below 50% of predicted values, MIP falls below −60 cm H_2O, or daytime $PaCO2_2$ increases above 45 mm Hg and the patient reports symptoms of orthopnea or symptomatic hypercapnia. New research on the timing of NPPV initiation suggests that these thresholds are too conservative and that patients may benefit from assisted ventilation when FVC drops to 65% of predicted values (Lechtzin et al., 2007). An earlier study by Melo et al. (1999) recommended that NPPV be offered to patients when FVC is less that 70% of predicted.

MIP appears to be a more sensitive measure of respiratory muscle weakness than FVC. In a retrospective study, all 161 ALS patients met U.S. CMS criteria for NPPV initiation with MIP −60 cm H_2O before FVC criteria of <50% of predicted. MIP criteria were reached 4 to 6.5 months earlier than FVC criteria (Mendoza et al., 2007). Obtaining MIP in addition to FVC on each clinic visit allows clinicians to obtain NPPV for patients with signs and symptoms of respiratory insufficiency, such as dyspnea and orthopnea. Conducting pulmonary function tests in the supine position is likely to produce lower FVC and MIP values than when patients are sitting upright. Supine pulmonary function tests are more likely to reflect nocturnal ventilation.

ACCEPTANCE OF NPPV

Much of what is known about patient acceptance of noninvasive assisted ventilation comes from sleep medicine and the treatment of OSA. Patients who are not symptomatic despite objective tests revealing pulmonary muscle weakness are less likely to use a device that is perceived as, at best, an inconvenience. Others will prefer to be proactive and embrace NPPV as well as other interventions (PEG tubes, speech augmentation devices, medication) in the hopes of managing symptoms and prolonging life. For some patients, accepting NPPV is accompanied by an acknowledgment that ALS is a terminal disease with respiratory failure the primary cause of death. Jackson et al. (2006) found that symptomatic orthopnea and dyspnea were the factors most closely associated with NPPV acceptance. Bourke et al. (2003) found of the five criteria for the initiation of NPPV, orthopnea was the best predictor of adherence to treatment as well as the best predictor of benefit.

Practice parameters recommend discussion of the disease course and treatment options to be held soon after diagnosis (Miller et al., 1999). Clinicians have a professional responsibility to provide patients and their families with the information necessary to make informed decisions about treatment options. Clinicians will certainly have their own professional opinions and personal biases regarding respiratory support and end-of-life decisions. It is imperative that patient independence, autonomy, and right to self-determination be respected.

ACCLIMATIZATION

Again, much of what we know about patients' ability to adjust to NPPV comes from sleep technologists, physiotherapists, and RCPs who work with OSA and its treatment with CPAP and bilevel positive airway pressure. Adjustment to positive pressure breathing is a process and involves psychological and physical adjustments. Desensitization is often necessary. A self-directed stepwise guide adapted from the University of Washington Medical Center's Northwest Assisted Breathing Center is summarized here (Boitano et al., 2007):

1. Wear interface (mask or nasal cushions) for 0.5 to 1 hour once or twice a day while not connected to the respiratory assistive device. Distract yourself by reading, listening to music, or watching television. Guided imagery and meditation may also be useful.
2. Attach interface to the respiratory assistive device. Turn the blower on. Use the unit for short periods during the day using one or more of the distractions listed previously. Holding the mask in place instead of using the straps may contribute to a feeling of control. Begin with 1 to 5 minutes and progress to 0.5 to 1 hour.
3. Try using the device for a nap during the day. Adjust the interface for comfort in all sleep positions you prefer—left side, right side, on your back.
4. Use the respiratory assistive device at night. If unable to fall asleep or awakening frequently, a prescription or over-the-counter sleep aid may be useful for the first week or two. If you awaken and

cannot fall back asleep with the device, remove it, and try again the next night. Do not skip a night. The more you use it, the easier it will become. Patients do not reap the benefits of use unless assisted ventilation is used at least 4 hours each night.

If patients are still having trouble falling asleep and staying asleep with NPPV, physicians may prescribe a sleep aid, antianxiety medication, or antidepressant with somnolent properties to use during the initial adjustment period.

ADHERENCE

Consistent use of NPPV over time varies with each patient and their adjustment to the device and their own disease progression. Severity of disease, degree of bulbar involvement, vital capacity, and general health status affect NPPV adherence/compliance (Jackson et al., 2006). Not only severity of symptoms but also symptom relief encourages continued use. Consistent follow-up by home care RCPs and multidisciplinary clinic staff for pressure adjustments to accommodate disease progression along with flexibility in offering a variety of interfaces will improve the ability of ALS patients to adhere to treatment.

Pinto et al. (2003) found that compliance with NPPV was significantly improved when treatment was initiated at the first objective sign of respiratory insufficiency. Nocturnal desaturation was used as a measure of early respiratory insufficiency, based on at least 15 desaturation events per hour (defined as a 4% drop in SpO_2 from baseline).

NPPV AND COGNITIVE IMPAIRMENT

Hypoventilation and hypoxemia can result in cognitive changes in ALS. Patients diagnosed with frontotemporal dementia have been shown to have lower FVCs (66%) than controls (99%) (Lomen-Hoerth et al., 2003). Lower FVCs may also contribute to lower scores in cognitive functioning, specifically memory retention, retrieval efficiency, and verbal fluency (Woolley, 2008).

The role of cognitive impairment on patient acceptance of treatment options in ALS is now being discussed (Woolley, 2008). In a retrospective cohort study at the University of California, San Francisco, Olney et al.

(2005) found that 75% of patients with frontotemporal dementia were noncompliant with NPPV compared with 38% of those who did not exhibit loss of cognitive and executive function.

NUTRITION AND NPPV

Registered dietitians are also concerned with increased work of breathing and energy expenditure with untreated respiratory insufficiency. Weight is followed closely and measured during each clinic visit. Weight loss is largely due to loss of muscle mass and poor oral intake; however, an increased metabolic rate with increased work of breathing and energy imbalance can lead to muscle catabolism for energy, further reducing muscle mass. NPPV during sleep and for fatigue during the day can aid nutritionists in managing caloric needs.

NPPV IN NEUROMUSCULAR DISEASE

Mode

Noninvasive positive pressure ventilators are designed to deliver PSV. The level of pressure support is the difference between IPAP and EPAP. The newer generations of NPPV allow IPAP pressures as high as 30 cm H_2O and EPAP settings as high as 15 cm H_2O. Returned tidal volumes need to be monitored and IPAP pressures increased as respiratory muscle and chest wall compliance decreases.

Portable home NPPV units had restricted patients to PSV mode. Volume-control ventilation became available in October 2007 with Respironics' BiPAP AVAPS (Murraysville, PA). With average volume-assured pressure support, tidal volumes are maintained by automatic adjustment in pressure. Other manufacturers are sure to follow suit with combined pressure and volume ventilation options for home use. Although designed with the neuromuscular patient in mind, the only crossover trial comparing NPPV in S/T mode with and without AVAPS has been conducted in patients with obesity hypoventilation syndrome (Storre, 2006). At this time, it appears that either PSV or VCV is capable of providing effective, well-tolerated NPPV to patients with neuromuscular disease (Chadda et al., 2004). Patient preference and respiratory symptom relief can guide choice of modality. A review of studies comparing NPPV modes in patients with chronic respiratory failure can be found in the August 2006 issue of *Respiratory Care* (Hess, 2006).

Apnea Backup Setting

Whether using PCV or VCV, spontaneously breathing neuromuscular patients should always use the S/T mode. Muscle weakness in ALS and a loss of the use of accessory muscles of respiration in REM stage sleep may result in an inability to trigger unit to inspiration. In addition, people with ALS may exhibit central apnea. For this reason, autotitration units should never be used in this patient population.

Cycle From Inspiration to Exhalation

Flow-cycling or time-cycling moves pressure delivery from IPAP to EPAP. In PSV in the spontaneously breathing patient, ventilation moves from end inspiration to exhalation when flow drops to a preset fraction of peak inspiratory flow (Hess, 2006). Flows are manipulated by setting an inspiratory time or an inspiratory time percentage. Mask leaks will alter the time of the inspiratory phase, causing patient discomfort and air trapping; however, NPPV units for home use are designed with a leak compensation feature. The amount of leak from a mask or nasal cushion system is factored into the algorithms of many NPPV units designed for the home-care market. Leaks are recorded and are available through data retrieval. Although lacking a true exhalation valve, with sufficient expiratory flow through the mask ($\geq$ EPAP 4 cm H_2O), CO_2 rebreathing is largely avoided.

Rise Time

Setting a rise time appropriate for the patient is key for patient comfort and acceptance of NPPV. Rise time determines how long it takes for the set inspiratory pressure to be reached, allowing for cycle to exhalation. In the absence of acute exacerbations or COPD, patients with ALS generally require a slower rise time.

Supplemental Oxygen

Because hypoxemia in ALS is generally due to ventilatory impairment and not an alveolar or parenchymal process, supplemental oxygen with NPPV is usually not necessary. Oxygen may be needed if patients develop an acute respiratory infection like pneumonia and a decrease in oxygen diffusion across the alveolar–pulmonary capillary membrane (increasing the A-a oxygen gradient). Respiratory assistive devices designed for home use lack an internal oxygen blender and therefore the capability of delivering a precise FIO_2. Oxygen can be bled into the NPPV circuit from an oxygen concentrator, liquid oxygen, or compressed gas system. Liter flow is titrated until the patient's oxygen saturation is more than 95%. Liter flow capabilities from home oxygen systems range from 1 to 6 liters per minutes (LPM) or 1 to 10 LPM, depending on the device, thus limiting FIO_2 capabilities to 0.40 to 0.60.

NPPV SETTING GUIDELINES

In most cases, beginning treatment with NPPV as soon as pulmonary function tests and patient-reported symptoms indicate hypoventilation allows clinicians to set IPAP and EPAP pressures in a low range. Pressure will be titrated upward as patients acclimate to assisted breathing. The following guidelines may assist RCPs with NPPV initiation.

1. Set Mode to S/T.
2. If using pressure-limited noninvasive ventilation, the initial setting of IPAP and EPAP should be 8 cm H_2O and EPAP of 4 cm H_2O, respectively, with IPAP adjusted for comfort.
3. Observe the patient's respiratory rate and breathing pattern (I:E ratio) and set backup rate to three to five breaths per minute below the resting respiratory rate. (Because hypoventilation will occur initially during sleep, NPPV settings should be titrated to patient comfort with patient lying flat or with the head of the bed slightly elevated if orthopnea is reported.)
4. Control inspiratory time by setting IPAP Max slightly longer than patient's inspiratory time and IPAP Min slightly shorter than patient's inspiratory time.
5. Alternately, set the rise time, inspiratory time, and I and E trigger sensitivity to meet patient ventilatory demands that allow for ventilator and patient synchrony. (Options will vary with the manufacturer and software.)
6. Tidal volumes should be monitored with a goal of 6 to 7.5 milliliter per kilogram of ideal body weight and IPAP pressures increased incrementally to achieve this goal.

7. Patients should be queried for signs and symptoms of nocturnal hypoventilation.

8. Nocturnal pulse oximetry can also be monitored if more objective measures are desired.

9. End-tidal CO_2 may be measured pre-NPPV trial and immediately after removing mask to ensure that patient is not underventilated or overventilated.

MONITORING NPPV SETTINGS

Most NPPV units designed for the home display and/or record tidal volumes achieved by IPAP/EPAP settings. The patient's respiratory rate and the percentage of patient-initiated breaths are also displayed, allowing clinicians to monitor patient response. Some NPPV units use a "smart card" system, allowing patients to mail the card to clinicians for data retrieval and review. Data can also be accessed remotely. In some cases, changes in settings can be made on the card for uploading into the NPPV unit when it is returned to the patient. Monitoring via telephone or cable lines may also be an option with some units. Personal computer software allows clinicians to adjust patient parameters directly from a computer monitor. Nocturnal SpO_2 and $ETCO_2$ may also be monitored to track oxygenation and ventilation status after initiation of NPPV and after pressure changes. This requires the patient to take home and return portable diagnostic units.

INITIATING NPPV IN ADVANCED ALS

Patients who begin use of NPPV late in the disease course may have difficulty adjusting to assisted ventilation. Adaptation to chronic respiratory failure caused by respiratory muscle weakness results in blunting of central chemoreceptors and an inability to reset the CO_2 threshold. In the absence of discomforting dyspnea, patients with compensated respiratory failure may have difficulty transitioning from volume replacement therapy to reduced volumes when breathing independently. Anecdotal reports of shortness of breath, sometimes lasting an hour of more, following morning discontinuance of nocturnal NPPV have been related by RCPs caring for ALS patients. Clinicians experienced with the COPD patient population observe similar situations when transitioning patients recovering from treatment for exacerbation of underlying lung disease and acute respiratory failure. Weaning from assisted ventilation to spontaneous breathing often results in dyspnea, tachycardia, tachypnea, and anxiety as patients readjust to their chronic, compensated, steady state of respiratory insufficiency.

CHALLENGES TO NPPV

Challenges to successful use of NPPV fall into three main categories: patient interface (mask leaks and skin irritation), rhinitis, and aerophagia.

Patient Interface

The variety of cushions used to join the patient and the pressure generating device—the interface—have grown in recent years, thanks again to the increase in patients treated for OSA. Logging onto any number of Internet sites devoted to the sale of CPAP devices and disposable supplies will reveal an array of nasal masks, oronasal masks, nasal pillow systems, hybridized nasal pillow and oral mask combinations, and total face masks. Finding a comfortable interface is key to acceptance of NPPV. Patients should be given a choice of interface in consultation with a clinician familiar with their benefits and drawbacks. It is not uncommon for patients to try two or more mask systems before finding one right for them. Patients may prefer using one type during the day and another for sleep. For example, nasal cushions that allow for wearing glasses and feel less restrictive can be used during the day, and switched to another style, like nasal or full face mask, at night.

Managing the Symptoms

Mask leaks and skin irritation are two of the most vexing challenges for NPPV users and clinicians. These problems originate from the same source: poor fit and improper adjustment.

Strapping a mask on too tightly may only worsen a leak. High-quality nongel masks are made with dual cushions. This design allows air from the pressure generator to fill the space between the cushions creating a soft seal. A mask adjusted too tightly will negate this feature.

Mouth leaks create another challenge. Weakened facial muscles combined with moderate-to-high IPAP pressures may cause air to leak out of the mouth during sleep. Persistent patient reports of dry mouth should alert clinicians to this possibility. Using a full face mask, total face mask, or nasal mask and a chin strap may solve this problem. Newer products, such as a lip seal system or dual-airway interface (nasal cushions/oral mask), may be of assistance. Clinicians are encouraged to view online sites that carry CPAP supplies for new products that may benefit patients. For patients and clinicians, where interfaces are concerned, a picture is worth a thousand words.

Skin abrasion and pressure sores, especially on the bridge of the nose, can be avoided by alternating nasal or full face mask with an alternative interface, like nasal cushions or total face mask. Breathable, hypoallergenic tape, such as Duoderm or HyTape, may be used between the bridge of the nose and mask. Again, overtightening the mask straps will contribute to pressure sores.

Redness, irritation, or pimples may occur where the mask touches the skin. In the absence of a reaction to mask materials, washing the face and keeping the pores clean may eliminate these problems. Redness from mild pressure should go away within 15 to 30 minutes after removing the mask in the morning. Older patients who are losing collagen may find it takes longer. Older, friable skin must be carefully watched for breakdown.

Rhinitis

A common challenge to NPPV use is nasal passage and sinus irritation. This is primarily caused by inadequate humidity of inspired air and high-velocity airflow through the nasal turbinate. Patients may report pain, burning, or bleeding. The purpose of the nose, other than providing us with one of five senses—olfactory—is to filter, warm, and humidify inspired gases. Nasal hairs filter the air we breathe. Blood vessels close to the surface warm the air. A thin layer of mucus adds humidity. In order to trap and dispose of inhaled dry aerosols—pollens, soot, dust—glands increase production of mucus which encapsulates the offending substances for better removal. Allergic reaction to pollens may create a histaminic response leading to mucosal edema. Increased mucus and swelling narrows the nasal passage further, contributing to greater turbulence and resistance to air flow from a respiratory assistive device. The nose may respond to decreased humidity by increasing production of serous fluid resulting in a "runny nose." These normal and healthy responses to irritation make initiation of nasal NPPV a challenge.

Managing the Symptoms

Most patients adjust to NPPV use over time; however, if allergic rhinitis is suspected, topical steroid nasal sprays can be prescribed. If not contraindicated, antihistamines and decongestants can be tried. Many patients manage nasal passage irritation successfully using over-the-counter saline irrigation solutions and moisturizing gels. Pollens and other aerosols can be flushed from the nose using a buffered saline solution before using NPPV. Coating the lining of the nose with a saline gel that includes aloe vera may improve humidity and comfort while the nasal mucosa adapts to increased airflow.

In OSA, heated humidification has been associated with fewer symptoms attributed to the upper airway, such as dry nose, dry mouth, and throat (Mador et al., 2005). Passover humidifiers with variable temperature settings can be added to any respiratory assistive device, and most units have integrated humidifier chambers; however, using heated humidifiers creates its own set of challenges. Fluctuation in ambient bedroom temperature may cause condensation to collect in corrugated connecting tubing. To avoid inadvertent and unpleasant nasal or oral lavage from condensation rainout, patients should be instructed to place their NPPV unit below the level of the mattress on a low bedside table or stool. Other techniques used by patients include placing corrugated tubing under the bedcovers and encasing tubing in an insulation sleeve. Sleeves can be made from batting material used in quilting, bubble wrap, or socks with feet removed or can be purchased from an online CPAP supply company.

Heated wire circuits have recently become available for home use with CPAP and bilevel positive airway pressure devices. Unfortunately, they must be purchased separately and may not be reimbursed by insurance. Several online sites often offer tips for new users as well as product information. Several sites are listed in the resources section.

Aerophagia

Patients may report discomfort from gas or bloating upon initiation of NPPV or when IPAP pressures are adjusted upward. Gastric insufflation is relatively uncommon in ALS because IPAP pressures are usually below 25 cm H_2O. Because the lower esophageal sphincter pressure is estimated to be between 25 and 33 cm H_2O, pressure at or below this level allows the sphincter to maintain a seal (Bach et al., 1993). If the sphincter has lost its tone or if patients have a history of gastroesophageal reflux disease (GERD), they will be at greater risk.

Managing Symptoms

Patients can avoid swallowing air by keeping their head and neck in a neutral position during sleep. If they must sleep in a semifowlers position, using a wedge instead of multiple pillows will keep the head from dropping forward. The head of the bed may be placed on blocks for elevation. As ALS progresses, a semielectric bed will make patient positioning easier.

For mild bloating or gas, simethicone can be used. If GERD is suspected, antacids should be prescribed. Increasing rise time and/or increasing number of timed breaths for apnea ventilation can reduce air swallowing in NPPV. Reducing IPAP pressure may be necessary.

Donning and Removing the Interface

Patients with upper-extremity weakness or hand weakness and loss of fine motor skills will have difficulty donning and removing an interface, especially nasal and full-face masks. This can contribute to anxiety and reluctance to use NPPV. Patients may be reluctant to awaken a bed partner or caregiver to assist them in the middle of the night. Some nasal cushion devices may be easier for this patient population to use because of the lack of tight fitting headgear. Clinicians should allow patients to practice placing, removing, and repositioning a selection of interface options. An occupational therapist may be consulted for suggestions and use of assistive devices. In all cases, clinician support, encouragement, and creativity will improve the chances of successful NPPV use.

THE BULBAR PATIENT

One of the greatest challenges to NPPV use in ALS is moderate to severe impairment of bulbar-innervated musculature. A study by Aboussouan et al. (1997) found that almost two thirds of patients who did not adjust to NPPV had impaired bulbar-innervated musculature. More recent studies have found poor bulbar muscle function to be a predictor of NPPV intolerance (Gruis, 2005). Because a loss of muscle tone in the oropharynx contributes to airflow restriction on forceful exhalation, patients with bulbar impairment perform poorly on pulmonary function tests. This leads to an underestimation of strength of their inspiratory muscles (Lyall et al., 2000) and a discrepancy between measures of respiratory muscle weakness and subjective symptoms of respiratory insufficiency.

Clinicians should proceed with caution when soliciting symptoms in patients with bulbar muscle impairment. For example, this group can have difficulty distinguishing the sensation of choking when lying flat from orthopnea (Bourke et al., 2006). Bulbar patients have difficulty managing saliva. Without medications to reduce saliva production or induce oral dryness, NPPV use will be difficult and may put patients at risk of choking or aspirating oral secretions. NPPV will be ineffective in the presence of glottic dysfunction or when the inability to protect the airway results in hypoxemia (Bach et al., 2004). If a patient is unable to clear secretions despite the use of cough augmentation or has recurrent pneumonia even with NPPV use, noninvasive ventilation is inappropriate (Benditt, 2006).

Poor QoL caused by sleep-related symptoms may be improved with the use of NPPV in bulbar patients; however, Bourke et al. (2006) found that patients with poor bulbar function tolerated NPPV only 3.8 hours per day compared with 9.3 hours per day for those with better bulbar function. In addition, patients with poor bulbar function were not able to tolerate IPAP pressures as high as those with better bulbar function. An inability to titration IPAP pressures upward as inspiratory muscles weaken will lead to underventilation and risk of hypoxemia. Further studies need to be undertaken in order to assess the role of NPPV in patients with moderate to severe bulbar impairment. For these patients, tracheostomy alone or tracheostomy with ventilation may be more successful in alleviating symptoms of hypoventilation and dyspnea (Aboussouan et al., 1997; Shneerson & Simonds, 2002).

SUMMARY

NPVV has been shown conclusively to alleviate symptoms of respiratory insufficiency in ALS (Heffernan et al., 2006; Miller et al., 1999) and can prolong survival in ALS patients able to tolerate it (Bourke et al., 2006). RCPs and others who manage respiratory symptoms face challenges in helping patients acclimate to use of this treatment. Adherence to treatment will improve with pressure settings that maximize ventilatory support and interfaces that allow for a degree of comfort. Consistent clinician follow-up, flexibility, and creativity will contribute to optimal patient adherence.

REFERENCES

Aboussouan LS, Khan SU, Meeker DP, et al. Effect of noninvasive positive-pressure ventilation on survival in amyotrophic lateral sclerosis. *Ann Intern Med* 1997; 127:450–453.

Aboussouan LS, Khan SU, Banerjee M, Arroliga AC, Mitsuoto H. Objective measures of the efficacy of noninvasive positive-pressure ventilation in amyotrophic lateral sclerosis. *Muscle Nerve* 2001;24:403–409.

American Association for Respiratory Care. Respiratory Care Journal Consensus Conference: non-invasive positive pressure ventilation. *Respir Care* 1997;47.

Bach JR. *Noninvasive Mechanical Ventilation.* Philadelphia: Hanley and Belfus; 2002.

Bach JR, Alba A, Mosher R, et al. Intermittent positive pressure ventilation via nasal access in the management of respiratory insufficiency. *Chest* 1987;92: 168–170.

Bach JR, Alba AS, Saporito LR. Intermittent positive pressure ventilation via the mouth as an alternative to tracheostomy for 257 ventilator users. *Chest* 1993;103: 174–182.

Bach JR, Bianchi C, Aufiero E. Oximetry and indications for tracheostomy for amyotrophic lateral sclerosis. *Chest* 2004;126:1502–1507.

Benditt JO. Full-time noninvasive ventilation: possible and desirable. *Respir Care* 2006;51:1005–1012.

Boitano L, Dobrozzi J, Hilsen M, et al. University of Washington Resource Manual for Noninvasive Mechanical Ventilation. University of Washington Medical Center/Department of Respiratory Care Services, 2007. Available at boitano@u.washington.edu.

Bourke SC, Bullock RE, Williams TL, Shaw PJ, Gibson GJ. Noninvasive ventilation in ALS: indications and effect on quality of life. *Neurology* 2003;61: 171–177.

Bourke SC, Tomlinson M, Williams TL, Bullock RE, Shaw PJ, Gibson GJ. Effects of noninvasive ventilation on survival and quality of life in patients with amyotrophic lateral sclerosis: a randomized controlled trial. *Lancet Neurol* 2006,5: 140–147.

Brochard L, Isabey D, Piquet J, et al. Reversal of acute exacerbation of chronic obstructive lung disease by inspiratory assistance with face mask. *N Engl J Med* 1990;323:1523–1530.

Chadda K, Clair B, Orlikowski D, et al. Pressure support versus assisted ventilation in neuromuscular disease. *Neurocrit Care* 2004;1:429–434.

Gruis KL, Brown DL, Schoennemann A, Zebarah VA, Feldmn EL. Predictors of noninvasive ventilation tolerance in patients with amyotrophic lateral sclerosis. *Muscle Nerve* 2005;32:808–811.

Heffernan C, Jenkinson C, Holmes T, et al. Management of respiration in MND/ ALS patients: an evidence based review. *Amyotrophic Lateral Sclerosis* 2006; 7:5–15.

Hess DR. Noninvasive ventilation in neuromuscular disease: equipment and application. *Respir Care* 2006;51:896–911.

Jackson CE, Lovitt S, Gowda N, Anderson F, Miller RG. Factors correlated with NPPV use in ALS. *Amyotrophic Lateral Sclerosis* 2006;7:80–85.

Kaplan JD, Schuster DP. Physiologic consequences of tracheal intubation. *Clin Chest Med* 1991;12:425–432.

Kleopa KA, Sherman M, Neal B, Romano GJ, Heiman-Patterson T. Bipap improves survival and rate of pulmonary function decline in patients with ALS. *J Neurol Sci* 1999;164:82–88.

Lechtzin N, Shade D, Clawson L, Wiener CM. Supramaximal inflation improves lung compliance in subjects with amyotrophic lateral sclerosis. *Chest* 2006;129: 1322–1329.

Lechtzin N, Scott Y, Busse AM, Clawson LL, Kimball R, Wiener CM. Early use of non-invasive positive pressure ventilation prolongs survival in subjects with ALS. *Amyotrophic Lateral Sclerosis* 2007;8:185–188.

Lo Coco D, Marchese S, Pesco MC, La Bella V, Piccoli F, Lo Coco A. Noninvasive positive-pressure ventilation in ALS: predictors of tolerance and survival. *Neurology* 2006;67:761–765.

Lomen-Hoerth C, Murphy J, Langmore S, et al. Are amyotrophic lateral sclerosis patients cognitively normal? *Neurology* 2003;60:1094–1097.

Lyall RA, Donaldson N, Polkey MI, et al. Respiratory muscle strength and ventilatory failure in amyotrophic lateral sclerosis. *Brain* 2000;124:2000– 2013.

Lyall RA, Donaldson N, Fleming T, et al. A prospective study of quality of life in ALS patients treated with noninvasive ventilation. *Neurology* 2001;57: 153–156.

Mador MJ, Krausz M, Pervez A, Pierce D, Braun M. Effect of heated humidification on compliance and quality of life in patients with sleep apnea using nasal continuous positive airway pressure. *Chest* 2005;128:2151–2158.

Mazzini L, Corra T, Zaccala M, Mora G, Del Piano M, Galante M. Percutaneous endoscopic gastrostomy and enteral nutrition in amyotrophic lateral sclerosis. *J Neurol* 1995;242:695–698.

Meduri G, Conoscenti C, Menashe P, Nair S. Noninvasive mask ventilation in patients with acute respiratory failure. *Chest* 1989;95:865–870.

Melo J, Homma A, Iturriaga E, Frierson L, et al. Pulmonary evaluation and prevalence of non-invasive ventilation in patients with amyotrophic lateral sclerosis: a multicentre survey and proposal of a pulmonary protocol. *J Neurol* 1999;169: 114–117.

Mendoza M, Gelinas DF, Moore DH, Miller RG. A comparison of maximal inspiratory pressure and forced vital capacity as potential criteria for initiating noninvasive ventilation in amyotrophic lateral sclerosis. *Amyotrophic Lateral Sclerosis* 2007;8:106–111.

Miller RG, Rosenberg JA, Gelinas DF, et al. Practice parameter: the care of the patient with amyotrophic lateral sclerosis (an evidence-based review): report of the Quality Standards Subcommittee of the American Academy of Neurology: ALS Practice Parameters Task Force. *Neurology* 1999;52:1311–1323.

Nava S, Ambrosino N, Clini E, et al. Noninvasive mechanical ventilation in the weaning of patients with respiratory failure due to chronic obstructive pulmonary disease: a randomized, controlled trial. *Ann Intern Med* 1998;128: 721–728.

Newsom-Davis IC, Lyall RA, et al. The effect of NIPPV on cognitive function in ALS: a prospective study. *J Neurol Neurosurg Psychiatry* 2001;71:482–487.

Olney RK, Murphy J, Forshew D, et al. The effects of executive and behavioral dysfunction on the course of ALS. *Neurology* 2005;65:1774–1777.

Pinto AC, de Carvalho M, Evangelista T, et al. Nocturnal pulse oximetry: a new approach to establish the appropriate time for non-invasive ventilation in ALS patients. *Amyotrophic Lateral Sclerosis Other Motor Neuron Dis* 2003;4: 31–35.

Pinto AC, Evangelista T, de Carvalho M, Alves MA, Sales Luis ML. Respiratory assistance with a non-invasive ventilator (Bipap) in MND/ALS patients: survival rates in a controlled trial. *J Neurol Sci* 1995;129(Suppl):19–26.

Rideau Y, Janoski LW, Grellet G. Respiratory function in the muscular dystrophies. *Muscle Nerve* 1981;4:155–164.

Rubenfeld GD. Study design in the evaluation of noninvasive positive pressure ventilation. Consensus Conference: nonivasive positive pressure ventilation. *Respir Care* 1997;41:443–449.

Shneerson JM, Simonds AK. Non-invasive ventilation for chest wall and neuromuscular disorders. *Eur Respir J* 2002;20:480–487.

Simonds AK, Muntoni F, Heather S, et al. Impact of nasal ventilation on survival in hypercapnic Duchenne muscular dystrophy. *Thorax* 1998;53:949–952.

Storre JH, Seuthe B, Fiechter, et al. Average volume-assured pressure support in obesity hypoventilation: a randomized crossover trial. *Chest* 2006; 130:815–821.

Udwadia ZF, Santis GK, Steven MH, Simonds AK. Nasal ventilation to facilitate weaning in patients with chronic respiratory insufficiency. *Thorax* 1992;47: 715–718.

Vitacca M, Barbano L, D'Anna S, et al. Comparison of five bilevel positive pressure ventilators in patients with chronic ventilatory failure: a physiologic study. *Chest* 2002;122:2105–2114.

Woolley S, Katz JS. Cognitive and Behavioral Impairment in ALS. *Phy Med Rehabil Clin N Am* 2008;19:607–617.

QUESTIONS FOR RESEARCH

1. Of the current NPPV options, pressure-limited or volume-targeted ventilation, which is best tolerated by patients with neuromuscular disease?

2. What role does NPPV have in reducing the signs of cognitive impairment in this subgroup of ALS patients?

3. What factors are most likely to contribute to compliance with NPPV in the ALS patient population?

4. Does NPPV use significantly improve the quality of life of patients with ALS?

CHAPTER 9

Tracheostomy and Mechanical Ventilation

CHAPTER OUTLINE

CASE HISTORY

Mrs. Albertson was a 74-year-old woman in relatively good health who was not cleared for cataract surgery because of complaints of difficulty swallowing and "something wrong with her voice." Evaluation by a neurologist and MRI resulted in the diagnosis of a small brainstem cerebral vascular accident. She was evaluated by a gastroenterologist a year later for increasing dysphagia and diagnosed with stricture/dysmotility likely secondary to her cerebral vascular accident. At this time, routine blood studies were normal. Mrs. Albertson had decreased appetite and had lost approximately 30 pounds. She was started on oral nutritional supplements, two cans daily, and her primary care physician referred her to a local neurologist; however, the family declined.

Six months later she was seen again by the neurologist and reported the following symptoms: difficulty swallowing, excess saliva sometimes and dry mouth other times, lack of energy, weight loss, unsteady on her feet, drooling, shortness of breath, and no appetite.

Physical examination included the following: weight, 110 pounds; height, 68 inches; blood pressure, 130/62; heart rate, 56; and respiratory rate, 12. She had mild facial weakness and limb strength 4 to 4+ arms and legs. Deep tendon reflexes were 2+ with no Hoffman or Babinski. Tongue was atrophic, slow moving, and fasciculating with no jaw jerk. Fasciculations were in both arms.

A diagnosis of possible amyotrophic lateral sclerosis (ALS) was discussed with the patient and her husband. They were given information on increasing calories as well as intervention with percutaneous endoscopic gastrostomy (PEG). She was scheduled for appointment with her gastroenterologist but did not keep this.

Mr. Albertson called the neurology clinic a month later to say his wife was "unable to eat at all." He was advised to bring Mrs. Albertson to the emergency department for an evaluation and probable admission for PEG placement.

In the emergency department, her vital signs were as follows: weight, 102; blood pressure, 143/9, heart rate, 103; respiratory rate, 18; temperature, 37°C; and O_2 saturation, 98% on 21% O_2.

During clinical evaluation Mrs. Albertson denied dyspnea at rest or on exertion. She acknowledged increased lassitude and decreased energy along with frequent nocturnal awakenings for

urination. She had difficulty clearing oral secretions and pro-
found dysarthria. The exam was also remarkable for mild weakness in the upper limbs. Her lungs were clear, but breath sounds
greatly diminished. Breathing was quiet with decreased lung
expansion. Accessory muscle use was not evident. She had never
smoked cigarettes or been exposed to hazardous fumes or dusts.
She had been a social drinker, but no longer drank alcoholic
beverages.

Initial labs were remarkable for HCO_3^- of 46, consistent with
compensated respiratory acidosis versus contraction alkalosis
with dehydration. She also had abnormal urinary analysis with
symptoms of a urinary tract infection and was started on
antibiotics.

Mrs. Albertson was admitted to the hospitalist service after
discussion with the gastroenterologist. Recommendations at
that time were hydration, oral hygiene and suctioning, schedul-
ing for PEG later in the week, swallow evaluation for safety,
nutrition consultation for supplement recommendations, and
a preoperative pulmonary function study. Code status and the
possibility of dependence on mechanical ventilation (MV) after
intubation were discussed. The patient and her husband wanted
"everything to be done" as long as there was a chance her status
could be improved with better nutrition.

On admission to the hospital, an "adult oximetry procedure"
order that included a standing order set; "check oxygen saturation and titrate oxygen to obtain saturation of 93% to 99%" was
put in place. That evening, Mrs. Albertson's oxygen saturation
was noted to be 88%. The covering physician was notified, and
Mrs. Albertson was started on oxygen at 1 L/min. Her oxygen
saturation increased to 94%. Pulmonary function tests and arterial blood gases were ordered for the following day.

The next morning, Mrs. Albertson had a dramatic change in
status.

Nursing Notes
06:40 no change, dysarthric
08:30 "hard to arouse, but then OK." Oxygen liter flow noted
to be 1.5 L/min

08:40 Oxygen increased to 2 L/min

09:30 Out of bed, in chair

11:00 "hard to arouse, ABGs drawn." Rapid response team called.

Initial ABGs: pH 7.12 PCO_2 136 PO_2 211 HCO_3 42.2 (11:36)

Subsequent ABGs following manual ventilation and subsequent noninvasive positive pressure ventilation (NPPV):

pH 7.33 PCO_2 77 PO_2 61 HCO_3 40.1 (14:02)

pH 7.38 PCO_2 66.3 PO_2 100 HCO_3 38.8 (16:41)

The following day a palliative care consultation was requested, and a do not resuscitate/do not intubate directive was discussed with patient and husband. No decision was reached.

ABGs results on 21%:

pH 7.38 PCO_2 65.9 PO_2 73 HCO_3 37.8

The next day, with Mrs. Albertson medically stable, a PEG procedure was performed. Oxygen saturations had decreased to 83% during the procedure in which Versed was administered. ABGs following procedure:

pH 7.28 PCO_2 96.9 PO_2 27 HCO_3 44.1

Mrs. Albertson was maintained on noninvasive positive pressure ventilation after PEG. She continued on NPPV for the next 2 days because of continued lethargy and was able to tolerate it up to several hours initially. As she became more alert, she refused to use assisted ventilation consistently, but was able and willing to tolerate it for short periods of time.

Three days later Mrs. Albertson again became unresponsive. Her husband was reached by phone, but no consensus was reached among family members regarding intubation and ventilation. A pulmonologist was called, and Mrs. Albertson was intubated and placed on MV.

Later, during a family conference, it was decided Mrs. Albertson would wish for comfort care only. She died shortly after extubation.

INTRODUCTION

Consistent use of noninvasive MV is able to improve gas exchange, lung compliance, and reverse nocturnal hypoventilation and chronic respiratory insufficiency in people with ALS. NPPV improves symptoms of respiratory insufficiency—exercise tolerance, dyspnea, sleep deprivation —and also improves speech volume and word generation (Bach, 2002). NPPV is able to increase survival time (Aboussan et al., 1997; Miller et al., 1999). As ALS progresses patients will become completely dependent on NPPV for ventilatory support. Because of the limits of IPAP pressures, typically 30 cm H_2O, NPPV may not be able to ventilate sufficiently patients with deteriorating lung compliance. At this point, patients must pursue hospice care or life support via tracheostomy and MV. Although MV will prolong survival, it will not affect the disease progression, and patients will become paralyzed. A minority of patients will progress to a "locked-in" state, unable to communicate. This chapter reviews predictors of whether patients will choose invasive MV in ALS, patient characteristics, caregiver responses, financial and social considerations, advantages and drawbacks, safety and mobility issues, and home MV models.

INDICATIONS FOR TRACHEOSTOMY AND MV

In ALS, the primary indications for tracheostomy and MV are failure of NPPV to relieve chronic respiratory insufficiency and acute respiratory failure. Inability to control the upper airway and risk of aspirating pooled saliva are contraindications to NPPV (Dotson et al., 2005). A subset of patients with moderate-to-severe bulbar symptoms may find that NPPV does not control their symptoms of hypoventilation (Borasio & Kaub-Wittemer, 2004). Refractory sialorrhea with inability to manage copious saliva makes NPPV difficult and may increase risk of aspiration. Patients who develop acute respiratory failure due to viral or bacterial pneumonia may opt for invasive ventilation temporarily in the hopes of being weaned to NPPV after the infection has resolved. The degree of diaphragmatic involvement determines weaning potential. Patients may have to undergo tracheostomy and maximize nutritional support as part of the road back to NPPV or mouthpiece ventilation.

Patients who are unable to be weaned from MV and have a progressive disease that requires increasing ventilatory support are eligible for long-term MV in the home. Failure to wean is defined by an inability to maintain ventilation ($PaCO_2 < 50$ mmHg) and inability to maintain oxygenation ($PaO_2 > 65$ mmHg with $FIO_2 < 30\%$) for at least 10 hours (Heffernan et al., 2006).

Elective tracheostomy is suggested for patients who cannot be adequately ventilated noninvasively. The hospital course is more likely to be shortened and uncomplicated with an elective procedure (Bach et al., 2004). Patients who delay a decision about hospice or tracheostomy and MV risk complications of acute respiratory failure and emergency intubation, including airway trauma, brain anoxia, and emotional distress.

The increased costs of emergency and critical care resulting from emergency tracheostomy can impose a financial hardship on patients with inadequate insurance coverage (Polkey et al., 1999). In the United States, between 5% and 8% of patients with ALS are placed on long-term MV, not all of them by choice (Bromberg, 2001). The ALS CARE database indicates that 3.2% of patients with ALS who have a forced vital capacity less than 40% of predicted were being treated with MV (Bradley et al., 2001). In one study, fewer than half of the patients with ALS maintained on MV had chosen this option in advance (Moss et al., 1996). A German study of 53 ALS patients receiving assisted ventilation found of the 21 patients on MV, 29% had not been informed in advance about the terminal nature of ALS and consequences of respiratory failure and 81% received tracheostomy without informed consent (Kaub-Wittemer et al., 2003).

ADVANTAGES OF TRACHEOSTOMY AND MV

Advantages of tracheostomy and invasive MV are preventing aspiration (pooled saliva, food boluses, and thin liquids), providing a more secure ventilator interface (tracheostomy tube connector versus mask), and ability to provide higher ventilator pressures (necessary as ALS progresses) (Andersen et al., 2005). The benefits of MV in ALS are similar to those of NPPV:

- Maintaining and/or improving oxygen/carbon dioxide levels
- Resting tired respiratory muscles

- Decreasing the work of breathing
- Improving chest expansion
- Improving sleep quality and avoidance of nocturnal hypo-ventilation
- Preventing/avoiding hospitalization for respiratory complications
- Improving quality of life (QoL)
  Adapted from Post-Polio Health International (2005).

The goals of tracheostomy and invasive MV are (1) to sustain and extend life, (2) to enhance the QoL, (3) to reduce morbidity, (4) to improve or sustain the physical and psychological function of the ventilator-assisted patient, and (5) to provide cost-effective care (American Association for Respiratory Care Clinical Practice Guideline, 2007).

DRAWBACKS TO TRACHEOSTOMY AND MV

Drawbacks to tracheostomy and invasive MV primarily result from potential complications of a long-term artificial airway and dependence on life support. Other drawbacks are the cost of supporting a patient on MV and the burden to family caregivers. These last two subjects are discussed in greater detail later in this chapter.

Potential Complications of Tracheostomy

- Increased secretions
- Mucus plugging
- Impaired swallowing
- Increased aspiration
- Increased risk of infection
- Tracheal eroding or tracheoesophageal fistula
- Tracheal stenosis or tracheomalacia

Potential Safety Issues of MV

- Accidental disconnection from the ventilator
- Malfunction of mechanical ventilator
- Unexpected decannulation
- Inadequate home electrical capabilities
- Illness or disability of primary caregivers

- High turnover of trained in-home nursing staff
- Poorly trained attendant care staff
- Difficulty and safety traveling to physician and clinic appointments

Home care-based respiratory care practitioners (RCPs) are knowledgeable about home safety and can offer practical solutions. Elective tracheostomy and advanced decision making allow family members to be trained in troubleshooting home mechanical ventilators and the cleaning and maintenance of tubing and respiratory equipment. Family members need time to develop the skills necessary to manage an artificial airway—tracheal suctioning, cleaning of the stoma site, changing the inner cannula, and replacing the tracheostomy tube.

MAKING THE DECISION FOR MV

Informed consent is only possible with patient education. ALS patients should be fully informed of the advantages and disadvantages of tracheostomy and MV. The ALS Association designed and published a series of manuals for patients and families, *Living with ALS.* Manual 6, *Adapting to Breathing Changes*, lists six questions to guide patient decision for long-term MV (Oppenheimer, 2002):

- Is it advised by your doctors?
- Is it desired by you and your family?
- Do you have the necessary resources available, including caregivers' help?
- Are you, your family, and/or friends able to learn the needed skills?
- Can you afford the cost of long-term invasive ventilation?
- Would you be able to live at home or need to be in a nursing home?

Physicians working closely with ALS patients emphasize that the decision to accept or reject MV is highly personal. It is based on practical considerations, the impact on friends and family, and perceptions of improved or reduced QoL. The decision should be made well in advance of severe respiratory compromise.

CHARACTERISTICS OF PATIENTS WHO CHOOSE MV

Characteristics of patient who choose tracheostomy and MV to treat respiratory failure include younger age and children under the age of 21 (Rabkin et al., 2006), higher levels of optimism, and overall life satisfaction. Patients who choose MV have more positive appraisals of their physical health and ability to function in daily life (Rabkin et al.).

Characteristics that favor a positive outcome after tracheostomy and home-based MV include the following (Gelinas, 2000; Rabkin et al., 2006):

- Slowly progressing ALS
- Highly motivated patient who is engaged in living
- A thorough understanding of the options
- The ability to communicate
- The ability to perform some activities of daily living
- A family willing and able to support MV
- The financial resources for medical equipment and in-home caregiver support
- An experienced multidisciplinary team that supports home ventilation

MEASURING QoL

QoL of ALS patients and their caregivers has received more attention over the past 10 years (Gelinas et al., 1998; Jenkinson et al., 2000). The World Health Organization (2000) defines QoL as "a broad ranging concept affected in a complex way by the person's physical health, psychological state, level of independence, social relationships, personal beliefs and their relationship to salient features of their environment."

To determine QoL of ALS patients and caregivers researchers measure health status (physical, functional, emotional, and mental well-being) and non–health-related factors (jobs, family and friends, religion and spirituality, coping, intimacy, desires, and goals) (Simmons et al., 2006). Researchers have used a variety of QoL assessment tools to study the lives of mechanically ventilated ALS patients and their primary caregivers, making study comparisons difficult (Bromberg & Forshew, 2002). Most QoL instruments link overall QoL with health status. Patient-perceived QoL in ALS does not correlate with physical function (Simmons et al., 2000). Life-prolonging interventions in ALS may not necessarily improve QoL. A validated disease-specific QoL instrument for ALS emphasizing the importance of nonphysical factors was recently published (Simmons et al., 2006). Consistency in measurement of QoL in ALS will increase the understanding of the breadth of factors influencing health and well-being in patients and their loved ones and will assist researchers in determining the benefits of interventions on patients' lives.

CHALLENGES OF MV

Financial

The financial cost of managing a patient at home on MV is great, up to $200,000 per year. Nursing care is typically not covered by insurance in the United States, and families must pay for the cost out of pocket (Rabkin et al., 2006). Paid caregivers, particularly nurses, are the most expensive component of home health care and can run as high as $250 per day.

Family finances affect choice of MV. In their prospective study of ALS patients who chose long-term MV, Rabkin et al. (2006) found annual household incomes above $100,000 to be a factor in choosing MV. Those without significant financial resources may find it cost prohibitive to care for a ventilator-dependent patient at home. If institutional care is chosen as an alternative to home care, finding a skilled nursing or subacute level of care with vacancies close to home may also be difficult. In Western Europe, financial considerations have not been noted as a primary issue in choosing MV because only a minority of patients incurs out-of-pocket expenses for home care (Borasio et al., 2001; Kaub-Wittemer et al., 2003).

Social workers in ALS clinics assist patients in examining medical benefits and personal and family assets. They can instruct the patient in how to apply for disability and other federal and state benefits and provide referrals to community resources for the patient and family. They can provide details of various levels of care from which to choose based on patient preference and options—skilled nursing care, subacute care, or home. The ALS Association and the Muscular Dystrophy Association, which also serves patients with ALS, offer an array of services and support.

Burdens of Caregiving

Caring for a person maintained on MV places substantial physical and psychological burdens on primary caregivers, typically spouses, partners, or adult children. A summary of caregiver responses to caring for ALS patients on MV follows:

- MV, even if initiated in an emergency situation without informed consent, seems to result in good generic QoL for patients, but at the price of a very high burden for their caregivers (Kaub-Wittemer et al., 2003).
- QoL and depression remained steady in patients with ALS, but caregivers experienced a significant increase in burden and depression after the patient was placed on MV (Gauthier et al., 2007).
- Patients often underestimate the burdens placed on those who care for them (Rabkin et al., 2006).
- QoL of patients and their caregivers are not interrelated. Couples do not represent a unique psychological entity, and their ability to cope with stressful and burdening situations is individual (Lo Coco et al., 2005).
- Caregivers report significantly higher physical and psychological burdens than their patients (Lo Coco et al., 2005).
- Forty-seven percent of caregivers said their own health had suffered (Moss et al., 1993).
- Forty-two percent of caregivers considered having the patient at home a major burden (Moss et al., 1996).
- Caregivers of MV patients report substantial levels of distress and were more likely to express regret about the decision for tracheostomy and invasive ventilation than the patient (Gelinas et al., 1998).
- Caregivers report substantial distress after initiation of MV despite having full-time aides (Rabkin et al., 2006).
- Caregivers who report lower QoL levels are not always those who have to look after the most physically or psychologically impaired patients (Lo Coco et al., 2005).

- Spirituality is not an important domain in QoL in MV and care of ALS patients at home (Lo Coco et al., 2005).
- Caregivers report their social activities outside the home are severely limited (Gelinas et al., 1998).
- Despite acknowledging the serious burdens, caregivers of ALS patients continue to report satisfaction with the caregiving role (Rabkin et al., 2006).
- Thirty percent of caregivers of MV/ALS patients rated their overall QoL lower than that of their patient and lower than the patient rated their own QoL (Kaub-Wittemer et al., 2003).
- Perceived burden was not found to be related to participation in support group or the number of substitute caregivers (Chio et al., 2005).
- Psychological stress (mood, burden, and strain) increased significantly in caregivers of ALS patients on MV (Goldstein et al., 2006).
- Caregiver distress can be predicted by negative social support and initial satisfaction in social relationships (Goldstein et al., 2006).
- Caregivers who report greater burden also report more depressive symptoms, although clinical depression is uncommon (Chio et al., 2005; Rabkin et al., 2006).
- When asked if they would advise MV to their patient again, 75% of caregiving spouses would do so. If faced with a decision to use MV themselves, only 50% would do so. By comparison, of patients using MV, 81% would choose MV again (Kaub-Wittemer et al., 2003).
- Caregivers that report the least stress are those who spend more time outside the home and are able to attend to their own needs without feeling guilty (Gelinas et al., 1998).

In general, stresses encountered by families of patients receiving MV are due to having less time for other family members, diminished social activities, presence of strangers in the home (nurses, therapists), loss of privacy, feeling tied to the machine, and an ambiguous future (DeVita & Hegde, 1995). Measuring the level of patient disability, impact of social and cultural environment, availability of medical support, and coping mechanisms of patients and caregivers will increase the understanding of the impact of MV in ALS. Any QoL measure needs to include the primary caregiver (Kaub-Wittemer et al., 2003). ALS caregivers should receive the same attention and emotional, psychological, and social support as the patients themselves (Lo Coco et al., 2005).

Stresses of Patients Receiving MV

Even though the majority of patients with ALS report general satisfaction with life on MV, they may encounter a range of stresses (DeVita & Hegde, 1995). These include the following:

- Feeling tied to the machine, dependency
- Infections: treatment, social isolation, activity restriction
- Inadequacy: cannot reach potential
- Social stigma: personal and by others
- Isolation: inability to participate
- Decreased involvement in recreational activities

MECHANICAL VENTILATORS FOR HOME USE

The choice of ventilator for home use should be based on the patient's specific respiratory needs (American Association for Respiratory Care, 2007). Ventilators must be dependable and easy for family and professional caregivers to operate.

A volume-cycled ventilator for home use can be used invasively or noninvasively for sip ventilation, using an angled mouthpiece during the day and mask during sleep. They can be used for breath stacking to improve expiratory flow and cough ability. Ventilators designed for home use include volume-cycled and pressure-cycled options. Modes include volume control, pressure control, pressure support, spontaneous, and assist/control. SIMV mode in portable, volume-cycled ventilators increases work of breathing.

Alarms contribute to safety. Ventilators may have internal batteries and/or have the capability to be powered by an external battery. Portability is a key feature. Size and weight allow ventilators designed for home use to be mounted on an electric wheelchair and wired to its battery. Positive end expiratory pressure (PEEP) may be internal or provided by a flow restrictor added to the external exhalation port. Options may include pressure support for patients who can breathe spontaneously.

The primary features of mechanical ventilators designed for home use and available in the United States are listed in Table 9-1.

Table 9-1 Volume/Pressure Cycled Ventilators

Volume Ventilators	Mode	Tidal Volume	Pressure/Flow Rate	Breath Rate	PEEP	Trigger	AC Voltage	Battery	Dimensions	Weight	Alarms
LP10 Puritan Bennett www.puritanbennett.com	Assist/control, SIMV, pressure cycle	100–2,200 ml	2–100 LPM	1–20 BPM		Pressure	110–240 V, 50/60 Hz	Internal, up to 1 hr External with 12 V battery	9.75" H × 14.5" W × 13.25" D	35 lbs	Low/high pressure, low battery, power failure, malfunction
Achieva Achieva PS Puritan Bennett www.puritanbennett.com	Assist/control, SIMV, CPAP, pressure support with PS model	50–2,200 ml	2–150 LPM	1–80 BPM		Flow/Pressure	100–240 V, 50/60 Hz. Universal AC input	Internal, 4 hrs External, 12 V	10.75" H × 13.30" W × 15.60" D	<32 lbs	Low/high pressure, apnea, setting error, power switch over, low power
HT50 Newport Medical Instruments www.ventilators.com	Assist/control, Volume control, SIMV, CPAP, PS	100–2,200 ml	Pressure control; 5–60 cm H$_2$O, Volume control, 1–100 cm H$_2$O	1–99 BPM	0–30 cm H$_2$O (leak compensated)	Pressure	110–240 V, 50/60/ 400 Hz	Internal, up to 10 hrs depending on features used External with 12–24 V battery. Newport Supplemental Power Pack (24 V): Adds 50% more use time to internal battery	10.63" H × 7.87" W × 10.24" D	15 lbs	High/low pressure, high/ low minute volume, high/ low PEEP, circuit occlusion, apnea, press control level not reached, line, battery low, battery empty, power switch over
LTV 800 Pulmonetic Systems, Inc. www.pulmonetic.com	Assist/control, SIMV, Spontaneous, Control	50–2,000 ml	10–100 LPM	0–80 BPM	0–20 cm H$_2$O	Pressure	90–250 V, 47/63 Hz	Internal, 1 hr External with 12 V battery, automobile cigarette lighter adapter option	3" H × 10" W × 12" D	12.85 lbs	Low/high pressure, empty/low battery, low minute ventilation, apnea, power failure, malfunction, disconnect

Model	Modes	Volume	Pressure	Rate	PEEP	Cycle	Power	Battery	Dimensions	Weight	Alarms
LTV 900 Pulmonetic Systems, Inc. www. pulmonetic.com	Assist/ control, SIMV, CPAP, VC, PS, Control	50–2,000 ml	Pressure support of 0–60 cm H₂O	0–80 BPM	0–20 cm H₂O	Flow	90–250 V, 47/63 Hz	Internal, 1 hr External with 12 V battery, automobile cigarette lighter adapter option	3" H × 10" W × 12" D	13.4 lbs	Low/high pressure, low/empty battery, power failure, malfunction, low minute ventilation, apnea, disconnect
LTV 950 Pulmonetic Systems, Inc. www. pulmonetic.com	Assist/ control, SIMV, CPAP, VC, PC, PS	50–2,000 mL	Pressure control 1–99 cm H₂O; Pressure support of 0–60 cm H₂O	0–80 BPM	0–20 cm H₂O	Flow	90–250 V, 47/63 Hz	Internal, 1 hr External with 12 V battery, automobile cigarette lighter adapter option	3" H × 10" W × 12" D	13.4 lbs	Low/high pressure, low/empty battery, power failure, malfunction, low minute ventilation, apnea, disconnect
PLV–100 Respironics, Inc. www. respironics.com	Assist/ control, SIMV Control	50–3,000 mL	10–120 LPM	2–35 BPM	0–20 cm H₂O	Pressure	120–240 V, 50/60 Hz,	Internal, 1 hr External with 12 V battery	9" H × 12.25" W × 12.25" D	28.2 lbs	Low/high pressure, apnea, low battery, power failure, malfunction
PLV–102b Respironics, Inc. www. respironics.com	Assist/ control, SIMV, Assist/ control + sigh Control	50–3,000 mL	10–120 LPM	2–35 BPM ± 0.5; 36–40 ± 2	0–20 cm H₂O	Pressure	120 V, 50/60 Hz, 220–240 V, 50/60 Hz	Internal, 1 hr External, 12 V	9" H × 12.25" W × 12.25" D	28.9 lbs	Low/high pressure, apnea, low battery, power failure, malfunction
TBird Legacy VIASYS Healthcare www. viasyshealthcare. com	Assist/ control, PC, PS, SIMV, CPAP	50–2,000 mL	1–60 cm H₂O	2–80 BPM	0–30 cm H₂O	Flow	100–240 V, 47/63 Hz	Internal, 25 minutes External with 12 V battery	12.6" W × 14" D × 13" H		Low/high pressure, malfunction, low minute ventilation

PREPARATION FOR HOSPITAL DISCHARGE AFTER TRACHEOSTOMY AND MV

The safe and effective discharge from hospital to home following tracheostomy and initiation of MV requires detailed preparation, family education, and training by hospital-based and home care RCPs, and support of other members of the patient care team. This process should not be rushed. Hospital discharge planners can facilitate a team conference at which a realistic time line for discharge will be established. The average time to discharge is 2 weeks for newly trached and mechanically ventilated patients (Kohorst, 2005). Ideally, family members should room in with the patient for at least 24 to 48 hours, providing all aspects of bedside care with RCP and nursing staff available for support. Competency of family members should be demonstrated and documented.

The roles of health professionals in home MV are as follows:

RCP: teaching, ventilator care, pulmonary therapy
Nurse: teaching, tracheostomy care, general nursing care
Social worker: psychological support, mobilization of resources
Physician: medical therapy, coordination of care

SUMMARY

If MV is chosen by patient and family and supported by the physician and other members of the multidisciplinary team, the outcome can be rewarding. Keys to successful home discharge are patient medical stability, an honest and detailed assessment of family finances, caregiver support systems, ability and willingness of family members to provide care, open communication among all parties, and planning by a dedicated multidisciplinary team of health care professionals (Kohorst, 2005). RCPs can play a key role by providing a realistic view of what artificial airway care and ventilator maintenance entails. Family education, training, and ongoing support are essential to a successful transition from hospital to home and avoidance of readmission for respiratory complications.

REFERENCES

Aboussan LS, Khan SU, Meeker DP, et al. Effect of non-invasive positive pressure ventilation on survival in amyotrophic lateral sclerosis. *Ann Intern Med* 1997;127: 450–453.

American Association for Respiratory Care. Clinical Practice Guideline: Long-term invasive mechanical ventilation in the home—2007 revision and update. *Respir Care* 2007;52:1056–1062.

Andersen PM, Borasio GD, Dengler R, et al. EFNS task force on management of amyotrophic lateral sclerosis: guidelines for diagnosing and clinical care of patients and relatives. *Eur J Neruol* 2005;12:921–938.

Bach JR. Noninvasive respiratory muscle aids and intervention goals. In Bach JR (ed.). *Noninvasive Mechanical Ventilation.* Philadelphia: Hanley and Belfus; 2002.

Bach J, Bianchi C, Aufiero E. Oximetry and indications for tracheostomy for amyotrophic lateral sclerosis. *Chest* 2004;126:1502–1507.

Borasio GD, Shaw PJ, Hardiman O, et al. Standards of palliative care for patient with amyotrophic lateral sclerosis: results of a European survey. *Amyotrophic Lateral Sclerosis Other Motor Neruon Dis* 2001;2:159–164.

Borasio GD, Kaub-Wittemer. Respiratory symptoms. In Voltz R, Bernat JL, Boracio GD, et al. (eds.). *Palliative Care in Neurology.* New York: Oxford University Press; 2004.

Bradley WG, Anderson F, Bromberg M, et al. Current management of ALS: comparison of the ALS CARE Database and the AAN Practice Parameter. *Neurology* 2001;57:500–504.

Bromberg MB. Life support: realities and dilemmas. In Mitsumoto H, Munsat T (eds.). *Amyotrophic Lateral Sclerosis: A Guide for Patients and Families.* New York: Demos; 2001.

Bromberg MB, Forshew DA. Comparison of instruments addressing quality of life in patients with ALS and their caregivers. *Neurology* 2002;58: 320–322.

Chio A, Gauthier A, Calvo A, et al. Caregiver burden and patients' perception of being a burden in ALS. *Neurology* 2005;64:1780–1782.

DeVita MA, Hegde S. Neuromuscular disorders. In Dantzker DR, Macintyre NR, Bakow ED (eds.). *Comprehensive Respiratory Care.* Philadelphia: W.B. Saunders Company; 1995.

Dotson RH, Daniel BM, Frank JA. General principles of managing a patient with respiratory failure. In George RB, Light RW, Matthay MA, Matthay RA (eds.). *Chest Medicine: Essentials of Pulmonary and Critical Care Medicine.* Philadelphia: Lippincott Williams & Wilkins; 2005.

Gauthier A, Vignola A, Calvo E, et al. A longitudinal study of quality of life on depression in patient/caregiver couples. *Neurology* 2007;68:923–926.

Gelinas DF. Amyotrophic lateral sclerosis and invasive ventilation. In Borasio GD, Walsh D (eds.). *Palliative Care in Amyotrophic Lateral Sclerosis.* New York: Oxford University Press; 2000.

Gelinas DF, O'Connor P, Miller RG. Quality of life for ventilator-dependent ALS patients and their caregivers. *J Neurol Sci* 1998;160(Suppl 1):S134–S136.

Goldstein LH, Atkins L, Landau S, et al. Predictors of psychological distress in careers of people with amyotrophic lateral sclerosis: a longitudinal study. *Psych Med* 2006;36:865–875.

Heffernan C, Jenkinson C, Holmes T, et al. Management of respiration in MND/ ALS patients: an evidence-based review. *Amyotrophic Lateral Sclerosis* 2006;7: 5–15.

Jenkinson C, Fitzpatrick R, Swash M, Peto VALS-HPS Steering Group. The ALS health profile study: quality of life of amyotrophic lateral sclerosis patients and careers in Europe. *J Neurol* 2000;247:835–840.

Kaub-Wittemer D, von Steinbuchel N, Wasner M. Quality of life and psychosocial issues in ventilated patients with amyotrophic lateral sclerosis and their caregivers. *J Pain Symptom Manage* 2003;26:890–896.

Kohorst J. Transitioning the ventilator-dependent patient from the hospital to home. *Medscape Pulmonary Med* 2005;9. Available at http://www.medscape.com/viewarticle/514735. Accessed July 11, 2008.

Lo Coco G, Lo Coco D, Cicero V, et al. Individual and health-related quality of life assessment in amyotrophic lateral sclerosis patients and their caregivers. *J Neurol Sci* 2005;238:11–17.

Miller RG, Rosenberg JA, Gelinas DF, et al. Practice parameter: the care of the patient with amyotrophic lateral sclerosis (an evidence-based review): report of the Quality Standards Subcommittee of the American Academy of Neurology: ALS Practice Parameters Task Force. Neurology 1999;52:1311–1323.

Moss AH, Casey P, Stocking CB, et al. Home ventilation for amyotrophic lateral sclerosis: outcomes, costs, and patient, family, and physician attitudes. *Neurology* 1993;43:438–443.

Moss AH, Oppenheimer EA, Casey P, et al. Patients with amyotrophic lateral sclerosis receiving long-term mechanical ventilation. *Chest* 1996;110: 249–255.

Oppenheimer EA. Living with ALS: adapting to breathing changes. *ALS Assoc* 2002:42–43.

Polkey MI, Lyall RA, Davidon AC, et al. Ethical and clinical issues in the use of home non-invasive mechanical ventilation for palliation of breathlessness in motor neuron disease. *Thorax* 1999;54:367–371.

Post-Polio Health International. Information about Ventilator Assisted Living 2005. Available at ventinfo@post-polio.org and www.post-polio.org/ivun. Physician direction by Krivickas LS and Oppenheimer EA.

Rabkin JG, Albert SM, Tider T, et al. Predictors and course of elective long-term mechanical ventilation: a prospective study of ALS patients. *Amyotrophic Lateral Sclerosis* 2006;7:86–95.

Simmons Z, Bremer BA, Robbins RA, et al. Quality of life in ALS depends on factors other than strength and physical function. *Neurology* 2000;55:388–392.

Simmons Z, Felgoise SH, Bremmer BA, et al. The ALSSQOL: balancing physical and nonphysical factors in assessing quality of life in ALS. *Neurology* 2006;67: 1659–1664.

World Health Organization. *Cancer Pain Relief and Palliative Care.* Geneva: World Health Organization; 2000.

10

Home Care of the Amyotrophic Lateral Sclerosis Patient

CHAPTER OUTLINE

INTRODUCTION

Caring for patients with respiratory and neuromuscular diseases in the home is a recognized specialty within the practice of respiratory care. The American Association for Respiratory Care hosts a specialty section, and the chair of the home care section informs members of medical and insurance regulatory decisions and guidelines, as well as other information of importance to respiratory care practitioners (RCPs) and the patients they manage in the community. Standards and practices for home respiratory care are reviewed, and the American Association for Respiratory Care publishes best practice guidelines in its journal, *Respiratory Care*, and makes them available on its website. Durable medical equipment (DME) and home medical equipment companies may choose to be accredited by the Joint Commission, whose published standards hold companies to a high level of patient safety. Insuring continuum of care throughout all levels of care continues to be a patient safety standard. This continuum extends into the home and community. When a patient with amyotrophic lateral sclerosis (ALS) is admitted to the hospital with acute respiratory failure or for an elective procedure (percutaneous endoscopic gastrostomy tube or tracheostomy tube placement), RCPs who work primarily in the hospital, the home, and the multidisciplinary neuromuscular clinic can work together to make the transition from hospital to home a safe and effective one.

Approximately two thirds of licensed RCPs work in the acute-care setting, and many may not be familiar with the respiratory equipment, procedures, rewards, and challenges of their colleagues who practice in the community. Physicians, nurses, RCPs, and other allied health professionals who work in ALS clinics may be unfamiliar with new challenges and frustrations presented by rapidly changing insurance reimbursement requirements and how they impact the lives of ALS patients. This chapter provides an overview of the management of patients with ALS who require noninvasive and invasive ventilation in the home.

CASE HISTORY

The decision by people with ALS to use assisted ventilation is a personal one and requires careful consideration. Patients who first use noninvasive ventilation may later face a decision about continuing ventilation via a tracheostomy and a volume ventilator. Unfortunately, if the tracheostomy is an emergency procedure, patients may find themselves on life support unexpectedly. Herb Ingram's experience with assisted ventilation and his view of his quality of life are described here.

Herb Ingram, 72 years old, was diagnosed with bulbar ALS in January 2000. His symptoms started with slurred speech and muscle twitches and progressed to difficulty with swallowing. He was mobile until spring of 2004 and in summer 2004 was able to stand for short periods of time with help. At that time, he was still using his hands on a limited basis and typed on a Light-WRITER communication device. He and his wife Jackie took a course in sign language; however, his signing ability declined, and it became difficult for him to sign his needs at night.

In the last quarter of 2004, he experienced severe bouts of choking and gagging on mucus. He tried using BiPAP and Cough Assist, but neither was successful because of ill-fitting masks. He and his wife were aware that a tracheostomy could help alleviate the choking problem and discussed that prospect with the ALS clinic. The clinic staff was not encouraging because of the long-term ramifications of a tracheostomy—prolonging life with progressive ALS leading to complete paralysis. Because he still had good limb mobility and was so uncomfortable with the heavy secretions, however, they were leaning toward the tracheostomy for suctioning, but not for ventilation.

Fate intervened. While hospitalized for an impacted bowel, he experienced such severe gagging that his pulmonologist ordered surgery for a tracheostomy. The tracheostomy eliminated the choking problem but introduced another—throat spasms. Initially these were frequent and severe, sometimes lasting for an hour. Initially mucus was suctioned up to 20 times per day, and each time the suctioning triggered the spasms. They learned that partial inflation of the trach tube cuff helped to prevent secretions from dropping past the trach and that coupled with Lorazepam drops squirted against his inner cheek helped to control the spasms. Spasms became infrequent and less arduous. The Cough Assist was effective in removing mucus from the airway and virtually eliminated suctioning.

In the hospital, he started using tracheostomy positive pressure ventilation at night to rest fatigued breathing muscles and continued that for the next year at home with the LP10 ventilator. He is certain that the trach and the ventilator prolonged his life and kept him comfortable. Eventually he became sufficiently short of breath that he needed to use the ventilator full time.

Herb and Jackie are fortunate to be covered by Medicare and supplemental insurance, although some equipment costs come out of their pocket. He is mobile in his electric wheelchair, but it is an older model. His large and cumbersome ventilator must be wheeled alongside the chair when Herb is out of the house, requiring two caregivers. The ventilator is reliable, and that is the most important issue for him. They have an excellent live-in aide that cares for Herb during the day. Jackie takes over at night and on weekends.

Quality of life issues continue to concern Herb and Jackie. He is still able to communicate and do the simple things he enjoys: watching television, working and playing at the computer, and visiting with family and friends. Their concerns lay with the future as ALS progresses. Ventilator use, although prolonging life, complicates that issue (© *Ventilator-Assisted Living* 2004, used with permission).

GOALS OF RESPIRATORY CARE IN THE HOME

The primary goal of RCPs caring for patients with ALS in the home is to provide respiratory support. ALS is a progressive disease, and the level of respiratory support will increase over time. Symptom relief and patient comfort are emphasized. Patient and family education is essential and ongoing. Prevention of hypoventilation, hypoxemia, atelectasis, and respiratory infection are accomplished through assisted ventilation and secretion mobilization. RCPs hope to assist patients in meeting their own goals of improved quality of life and time with their loved ones.

TYPES OF RESPIRATORY SUPPORT

Volume expansion and secretion mobilization are the primary types of support provided by RCPs to ALS patients at home. If the patient has a history of asthma or chronic obstructive pulmonary disease with a reactive airway component, patients and family members will be instructed in the use and benefits of aerosolized bronchodilator and/or corticosteroid therapy. A Cough Assist device may be prescribed when the patient has a significant reduction in peak cough flow. If breath stacking has been demonstrated by the RCP in the clinic, the technique will be reinforced by the home care RCP.

Noninvasive positive pressure ventilation (NPPV) used initially at night and intermittently during the day is needed continuously as the diaphragm and accessory muscles continue to weaken. If the patient opts for "sip" ventilation, a volume ventilator with pressure support option is ordered with an angled mouthpiece for use during the day and a mask for use at night. If severe bulbar dysfunction, frequent aspiration, inability to adjust to NPPV, or insufficiency of NPPV ($PCO_2 > 50$ mmHg and $PO_2 < 65$ mmHg) results in respiratory failure, the patient must choose between tracheostomy and mechanical ventilation or entering hospice care. Each stage of ALS will require the patient to adjust to new methods of ventilation and additional patient and family education. Increased dependence on assisted ventilation triggers emotional responses in the ALS patient and in family members.

NPPV

Insurance Requirements and Reimbursement

Patients with ALS are prescribed a respiratory assist device (RAD), in Medicare parlance, to deliver NPPV. Medicare requirements for reimbursement of RAD include the following conditions:

1. Documentation of a progressive neuromuscular disease or a severe thoracic cage abnormality, and
2. An ABG $PaCO_2 \geq 45$ mmHg while awake on the patient's usual FIO_2, or a sleep oximetry $\leq 88\%$ for a least 5 continuous minutes on the patient's usual FIO_2 or for progressive neuromuscular disease

(only) maximal inspiratory pressure > - 60 cm H_2O or forced vital capacity < 50% of predicted, and

3. Written documentation that COPD does not contribute significantly to the patient's pulmonary limitation.

Most third-party payers follow Medicare guidelines and will authorize reimbursement for NPPV if the patient meets the basic criteria mentioned previously. There are no written guidelines for secretion mobilization equipment. A Cough Assist, the Vest, or other device may be considered experimental or investigational, and insurance companies may accept or decline reimbursement on a case-by-case basis. ALS clinics may have to submit letters of medical necessity to insurance providers in order to obtain an authorization for medical equipment rental.

The Cough Assist is expensive for DME companies to purchase. Insurance reimbursement may not cover the purchase cost. It may be difficult for the ALS clinic RCP to locate a DME provider who stocks or is willing to purchase this type of secretion mobilization unit.

Patients with health insurance through a preferred provider or health maintenance organization will need to choose a DME company that is approved by their insurer. If the patient chooses to go "out of network," a co-payment will be required. Some insurance plans do not include a DME benefit, in which case the patient is responsible for renting or purchasing the medical equipment. Patients who rely on the federal government's Medicaid program for health insurance may have difficulty finding a DME company to serve them. Anecdotal reports of DME companies' unwillingness to provide medical equipment to patients covered solely by Medicaid are increasing. As payment rates by Medicaid have decreased, home care companies find the cost of providing service is not met by federal and state government reimbursement.

In April 2006, Medicare changed the classification of RADs, no longer designating them DME requiring frequent and substantial servicing. RADs are rented for 13 months (rent-to-own), at which time they become the property of the patient. The patient becomes solely responsible for service and maintenance. Disposable supplies (tubing, filters, and masks) continue to be reimbursed.

Services of RCPs are not covered under the Medicare DME benefit. Only the monthly rental charge is reimbursed. DME companies had bundled monthly reimbursement for RAD rental with the services of

RCPs to monitor equipment and make setting changes in the home. Appeals to the Centers for Medicare and Medicaid Services from respiratory care professionals and organizations for people with neuromuscular diseases to reclassify RADs as DME have been denied.

Prescription

The prescription for NPPV includes IPAP and EPAP pressures and backup respiratory rate settings. The RCP in the ALS clinic determines the initial settings during the patient's clinic appointment. The prescription includes NPPV pressure ranges so the home care RCP can titrate settings for patient comfort as the disease progresses. Targeted tidal volumes and nocturnal SpO_2 may be used to titrate the IPAP pressure.

Initial Setup

The initial home visit involves a clinical assessment of the patient's respiratory status, ventilation requirements, and goals of therapy. A crucial and often time-consuming aspect of the visit is fitting the patient with an interface (nasal cushions, nasal mask, full face mask, or total face mask) that is comfortable and adjusted properly to avoid leaks and skin abrasions. The RCP conducts a brief trial of NPPV with the patient and makes pressure adjustments for comfort. Tips for acclimating to the device are offered. Proper functioning and maintenance of the NPPV and heated humidifier unit are covered. Maintenance includes filter cleaning, disinfecting tubing and interface (mask or nasal cushions), and ordering of additional disposable supplies. Contact information for the home care company and RCP is given, and a follow-up schedule is reviewed. A summary of the initial visit is sent to the ALS clinic and a copy placed in the patient's file.

Follow-up

RCPs make a follow-up phone call within the next few days. Patients with dysarthria may prefer to communicate by e-mail. A second home visit is scheduled. Fine-tuning adjustments are made for comfort (rise time, sensitivity, inspiratory time, and maximum inspiratory and expiratory pressures). After the patient is able to use NPPV consistently, at least 4 hours each night, exhaled tidal volumes can be monitored (data download) and settings modified. NPPV use and maintenance are reviewed with the patient and family. The interface is adjusted and replaced if necessary. An overnight oximetry study may be prescribed by the referring ALS clinic to monitor patient response to assisted ventilation. If the patient appears stable and pressure settings are adequate, home visits can be spaced further apart. Phone or e-mail check in with patient and family will assure consistency of care.

Continuous NPPV

The patient's respiratory status will eventually progress to the point where he or she requires noninvasive ventilatory support 20 to 24 hours a day. For patients without significant sialorrhea or difficulty protecting the airway, this expansion in respiratory care may be a smooth one. Using a variety of interfaces will increase comfort, for example, nasal cushions during the day and a mask at night. This will reduce continuous pressure on the bridge of the nose, where skin breakdown is most likely to occur. An interface that is easy to don and remove independently is ideal. Allowing time for patients to practice with an interface is helpful and increases confidence. A direct current adaptor will allow the NPPV unit to be powered by an electric wheelchair battery, giving the patient mobility within and outside the home.

TRACHEOSTOMY AND MECHANICAL VENTILATION

ALS patients and families who choose long-term mechanical ventilation will find advantages over NPPV: they will not risk respiratory failure if the interface is inadvertently removed, ventilatory support is improved, breath stacking is available, and a second unit is covered by insurance if used differently (one for bedside and one mounted on a wheelchair for mobility).

Home care ventilator options include those with volume-cycled/ pressure-control modes and pressure support (billing code E0646) and volume-cycled ventilators without pressure support (billing code E0461). Choice should be made based on patient's clinical needs, ability to trigger to inspiration, ability to breath stack, and comfort. Ventilators with volume control/pressure control and pressure support settings are more expensive and medical justification may need to be offered.

Discharge Plan

After tracheostomy and adjustment to mechanical ventilation in the hospital, a plan of care is developed by the multidisciplinary team and reviewed and signed by the physician. Adequate time is allotted to ensure tracheostomy has matured and healed. Sufficient time for family caregiver training in ventilator management and tracheostomy care must be allowed. The physician and social worker will confirm that it is the patient's choice to receive home mechanical ventilation before hospital discharge.

Home Environment and Safety Considerations

As part of the home discharge process and as a prerequisite for acceptance by the DME company, a RCP will visit the patient's home to assure patient safely. The home environment must meet basic requirements:

- Electrical safety. Grounded electrical outlets and sufficient number of outlets to accommodate ventilators, suction unit, sufficient lighting, and any other equipment needed in the bedroom. Adequate amperage to accommodate all medical equipment and household appliances.
- Functioning phone lines to contact and be contacted by emergency medical personnel.
- Uncluttered environment. Sufficient room in hallways and rooms to accommodate wheelchair and gurney, if emergency medical personnel are called to the home.
- No fire hazards. Presence of working smoke alarms and fire extinguishers.
- Clean and sanitary conditions. Space to clean, disinfect, and dry ventilator tubing and supplies if using nondisposable circuits.
- Air conditioning in warm climates. Electrical fans. Safe and efficient heating system in cold climates.
- Marine batteries or other source of direct current power available for unplanned long term electrical outages.
- If frequent power outages occur, possibly a portable generator.
- Easy access to the house by emergency vehicles. Uncluttered driveway, free space in front of house.
- A count of the number of stairs into and inside the home.

(*Respiratory Care*, 2007)

Infection Control

RCPs educate family caregivers about the risk of transmitting bacteria between patient and caregiver. Careful hand washing is emphasized, along with the appropriate use of gloves and disposal of medical waste. Family members are encouraged to get vaccinated against influenza and to minimize the patient's exposure to family members and visitors with upper-respiratory infections.

As part of education and training by the RCP, caregivers must be able to change the ventilator circuit without contaminating connections. Cleaning and disinfection of reusable ventilator circuits, passover humidifiers, and trach tube connectors must be done in a dedicated place within the home. Disposable supplies are stored in a clean, dry area. A designated area for tracheostomy cleaning supplies and disposable inner cannulas is established. Caregivers must demonstrate competency in cleaning nondisposable supplies before hospital discharge. The RCP will observe and monitor the caregiver technique and make suggestions after the patient has arrived at home.

General Safety Recommendations

When the ALS patient returns home on mechanical ventilation, the RCP can make recommendations to assist the family with general safety. Useful suggestions include the following:

- Ensure that the house location is clearly marked. Make sure that house numbers are large (at least 3 inches), well lit, and easy to see by emergency medical personnel.
- Prominently post important phone numbers with easy access to patient and phone (local fire department, police department, emergency medical response, physicians, home care RCP, and family members).
- Keep manual resuscitation bag at the bedside, and ensure that all caregivers are trained in its use.
- Keep a replacement tracheostomy tube of correct size and type at the bedside.
- Send letters to the telephone and electric power company, and ask that the house be placed on the emergency reconnect list in case of outages.

- Notify emergency management teams (fire, police, EMT) of the ALS patient at home on life support in case a call is made for assistance.
- Ensure that ventilator audible alarms are loud enough to be heard by caregivers in all areas of the home. Remote alarms (or baby monitors) can be used if alarm volumes are insufficient.
- Ensure that patients are able to summon caregivers to the bedside as needed. Call chimes can be adapted for use even when patient has little movement.

Ventilator Setup and Monitoring

When the patient arrives home from the hospital, the RCP will be there to assess proper functioning of equipment, patient's physical condition, and respiratory response to ventilation. Ventilation and alarm settings will be documented in the patient's chart. In addition to the ventilator settings, the RCP will check filters for cleanliness and document the power levels (charge) of the internal and external backup battery sources. The frequency at which the ventilator will be monitored by the RCP should be specified in the plan of care signed by the physician. Typically, the RCP will make home visits frequently in the first weeks after discharge. After the first 3 months, routine patient assessment and equipment maintenance are scheduled quarterly. The ventilator is scheduled for preventive maintenance once a year.

The RCP provides in-service training to in-home nursing and nonprofessional staff who assist family caregivers in ventilator maintenance and airway care. Family members are encouraged to contact the RCP with questions between quarterly visits to ensure patient safety and their own peace of mind. As ALS continues its relentless course, empathy and kindness become as valuable a resource as clinical knowledge.

CHALLENGES OF MANAGING MECHANICALLY VENTILATED PATIENTS IN THE HOME

In the Spring of 2006, the International Ventilator Users Network invited an international group of health care professionals to respond to this question: What are the major issues facing you as a health professional in treating/managing your patients who are users of home mechanical ventilation (*Ventilator Assisted Living*, 2006) Insurance reimbursement and obtaining medical equipment were the most common responses. Medical care of ALS patients in the home cannot be separated from the realities of the health care delivery system in the United States and abroad. In their own words, responses of physicians and RCPs follow:

> For me, the predominant issue is obtaining the funding for patients to receive appropriate care in the home. We have the technologies available to help people live longer and with better quality of life but appropriate coverage is shrinking. (Joshua Benditt, MD, FCCP, University Medical Center, Seattle, Washington)
>
> The Medicare guidelines for timely initiation of NPPV are restrictive. Payer support for mechanical ventilation and cough augmentation therapy is often difficult to obtain. Insurers are often resistant to supporting the newer generation of compact ventilators that allow for greater patient mobility with power wheelchairs. (Louis Boitano, MS, RRT, RPFT, University Medical Center, Seattle, Washington)
>
> I have patients who need Cough Assist units who cannot get coverage and inpatient respiratory therapists who just don't seem to 'get it' with regards to its benefits. Congress needs to pass Medicare guidelines that will allow separate billing for respiratory visits to the home, just like for nursing and PT/OT visits. (Brenda Jo Butka, MD, FCCP, Vanderbilt Stallworth Rehabilitation Hospital, Nashville, Tennessee)
>
> From the reimbursement standpoint—as competitive bidding and how to devise home care service to vent users when there is no provision to do so. It would be nice to have a template for standards of care to deliver home ventilator care that is updated and accepted for reimbursement. (Peter Gay, MD, FCCP, Mayo Clinic/Rochester, Rochester, Minnesota)
>
> A negative view of the outlook and prognosis in individuals with severe neuromuscular disease held by the public and health care professionals who are not routinely involved in their care, an assumption that one plan of medical management suits all, and a constant struggle to get funding—for research and ventilatory equipment. (Anita Simonds, MD, FRCP, Royal Brompton & Harefield NHS Trust, London, England)
>
> Getting insurance companies to understand that we no longer use 1990s technology. Dealing with discharge planners who want the patient to go home "tomorrow." Getting paid appropriately for the services we provide, such as training, which is paramount to living at home. (John A. Widder, BA, CRT, Los Niños Hospital, Phoenix, Arizona)

REFERENCES

The section *Tracheostomy and Mechanical Ventilation* is adapted from the
AARC Clinical Practice Guideline: Long-term invasive mechanical ventilation in the
    home—2007 Revision and Update. *Respir Care* 2007;52:1056–1062.

Ventilator Assisted Living. IVUN's New Medical Advisory Committee Shares its
    Views. 2006;20:4–5. Available at www.post-polio.org/ivun.

Ventilator Assisted Living. Quality of life: profiles of living with ALS. 2004;18:
    1–6.

11

Palliative Care and End-of-Life Care

CHAPTER OUTLINE

INTRODUCTION

Palliative care is an integral part of the continuum of care for patients with amyotrophic lateral sclerosis (ALS). Palliative care is well suited to the interdisciplinary team model that emphasizes treating the whole person within the context of their social support system. It is the model for care in ALS and is recommended by the American Academy of Neurology practice parameter (Miller et al., 1999).

Because there is no cure for ALS, in essence, all care is palliative. The emphasis is on patient comfort and symptom control. Most patients die of progressive restrictive lung disease and respiratory failure. Respiratory care practitioners (RCPs) are able to improve patients' quality of life (QoL) by assessing and managing the symptoms of respiratory insufficiency.

Dyspnea is one of the most distressing symptoms in ALS (Voltz & Borasio, 1997). When and how dyspnea occurs and the degree of its severity guide treatment recommendations. Breath is life. When patients are unable to maintain adequate ventilation independently, education about end-of-life options must be provided with the assurance that talking about death does not mean giving up on life.

The American Academy of Neurology and the American College of Chest Physicians have published position statements and guidelines emphasizing the importance of palliative care for patients with neuromuscular diseases. The American Association for Respiratory Care devoted two issues of *Respiratory Care* to end-of-life issues in respiratory disease (Respiratory Care, 2000). Physicians in the United States can now become certified in palliative care through the American Board of Hospice and Palliative Care. There is growing recognition that palliative care should be integrated into allied health and respiratory therapy programs.

Definition

Palliative care is the management of patients with progressive, life-threatening disease for whom the prognosis is limited. The 2002 World Health Organization defines palliative care as follows:

> An approach which improves quality of life for patients and their families facing life threatening illness through the prevention and relief of suffering by means of early identification and impeccable assessment and treatment of pain and other problems, physical, psychosocial and spiritual.

Holistic Approach

ALS requires a holistic, integrated approach to care that addresses all aspects of life: the physical (comfort and symptom control), emotional (fears and concerns), intellectual (information and education), social (family and friends), and spiritual (life review, meaning of life, and being at peace at the end of life). Support of patient and family is central, and patient autonomy must be respected at all times.

The tenets of palliation in life-limiting disease are summarized here (World Health Organization, 2002):

- Provides relief from pain and distressing symptoms
- Affirms life and regards dying as a normal process
- Intends neither to hasten nor postpone death
- Integrates the psychological and spiritual aspects of patient care
- Offers a support system to help the family
- Uses a team approach to address the needs of patients and their families, including bereavement counseling, if indicated
- Will enhance QoL and may also positively influence the course of the illness
- Is applicable early in the course of the illness

END-OF-LIFE CHOICES

Timing of End-of-Life Discussions

There are no standards for when and how end of life issues should be discussed with people diagnosed with ALS. The approach to end-of-life care in neuromuscular diseases is based on consensus of experts in ALS care and informed by the large body of literature for cancer and human immunodeficiency virus/acquired immune deficiency syndrome (HIV/ AIDS). Evidence-based literature reviews of end-of-life discussions in ALS have been conducted in the United States and Europe. Based on extensive research, good practice points on communicating the diagnosis of ALS and its implications have been published (Andersen et al., 2005; Heffernan et al., 2006; Miller et al., 1999). These recommendations are summarized here:

- The diagnosis of ALS should be pursued as early as possible. Patients in whom ALS is suspected should be referred with high priority to an experienced neurologist (Andersen et al., 2005).
- After a diagnosis has been made, the physician should give the diagnosis to the patient in person and discuss its implications in a stepwise fashion, allowing enough time (at least 45 to 60 minutes) . . . for questions (Andersen et al., 2005; Miller et al., 1999).
- Delivery of information must take into consideration the cultural and social background of the patient by asking whether the patient wishes to receive the information or that the information be communicated to a designated family member (Andersen et al., 2005; Heffernan et al., 2006; Miller et al., 1999).
- Initiate discussions on end of life decisions whenever the patient asks—or "opens the door"—for end of life information and/or interventions (Andersen et al., 2005).
- Initiate discussions about all treatment options such as noninvasive, invasive ventilation, and terminal phase as soon as symptoms or signs of respiratory problems develop to enable advance planning or directives (Andersen et al., 2005; Heffernan et al., 2006).
- Helping patients understand the issues to be faced in the terminal phase of the disease must be accomplished in a timely and empathetic fashion (Miller et al., 1999).
- Patients and families need information that is timed appropriately for decision making and delivered well in advance of major management crossroads, especially for respiratory care (Miller et al., 1999).
- The physician should introduce the discussions regarding advanced directives (ADs) and naming of a health care proxy and assistance

offered in formulating an AD (Andersen et al., 2005; Miller et al., 1999).

- Patients' wishes regarding their care and ADs should be reviewed regularly . . . at intervals of no more than 6 months (Heffernan et al., 2006; Miller et al., 1999).

Respiratory insufficiency and impaired ventilatory function usually occur later in the disease course but may be the presenting symptom or occur shortly after the onset of symptoms (Heffernan et al., 2006). The degree of respiratory impairment increases with the progression of ALS. Acute respiratory failure with unplanned emergency intubation and mechanical ventilation when the patient has not had the opportunity to make his or her wishes known is to be avoided (Kaub-Wittemer et al., 2003). For this reason, end-of-life decisions are encouraged early in the disease course, and do-not-resuscitate (DNR), do-not-intubate (DNI), or full ventilatory support choice should be documented in the patients' charts.

Studies of the specific timing of DNR/DNI discussions are lacking. To address this deficit, Munroe et al. (2007) conducted a retrospective analysis of 42 patients with ALS seen by neurologists and pulmonologists in one neuromuscular clinic. Physicians initiated end-of-life discussions with 95% of patients on the first visit. Two additional patients discussed end-of-life on the second visit. The most important factor in whether an ALS patient made a decision about resuscitation and ventilation was whether the physician addressed the issue in a timely manner. Factors with little bearing on patients' decisions were severity of lung disease as measured by forced vital capacity, bulbar dysfunction, and time from symptom development to definitive diagnosis.

There is a range of expertise among neurologists in palliative care and comfort with discussing the dying process (Maddocks, 2004). In general, physicians have difficulty talking about death and have not received training in how to communicate terminal diagnoses (Christakis, 1999). In his book *A Death Foretold: Prophecy and Prognosis in Medical Care*, British physician and sociologist Nicolas Christakis noted that there are three questions asked by patients with life-threatening illnesses that highlight the tasks expected of physicians: Why am I so weak? What can you do for me? Am I going to die? This last question is the most difficult to address with the patient. An inability to give a definitive prognosis can lead physicians to avoid discussion of death. If patients do not have accurate information regarding their prognosis, they may choose futile life-prolonging treatments over feasible palliative care (Weeks et al., 1998).

Patients with ALS generally welcome the opportunity to discuss end-of-life issues with their physicians (Benditt et al., 2001; Munroe et al., 2007; Silverstein et al., 1991). In the Munroe study, 83% of patients made a decision for DNI during their initial visit, suggesting that they had already given the issue much thought. In an end-of-life survey conduced by the California Healthcare Foundation, 80% of participants said that loved ones "know exactly" or have a "good idea" of what their wishes would be if they were in a persistent coma, but only 50% had talked to their loved ones about their preferences. Of the 50% who had spoken to loved ones about end-of-life wishes, 19% of the conversations were "casual," or remarks made in passing (November 2006); however, 74% to 89% of participants reported being "very" or "somewhat" comfortable talking about death. As healthcare providers, acknowledging and working out our own discomfort with discussing death and dying will help us to discuss these issues with patients who may look to us to open the lines of communication.

Education and Decision Making in ALS

Improved lung expansion and oxygenation through invasive volume ventilation and noninvasive positive pressure ventilation and improved nutrition through percutaneous endoscopic gastrostomy tube placement have increased life expectancy in people with ALS. ALS progresses gradually and is individualized. Each stage brings with it new decisions, information, medical equipment, and challenges. Patients' choices about end-of-life care may change over time, and thus, opportunities to discuss end-of-life decisions should be offered at each quarterly clinic visit (Albert et al., 1999). A decline in respiratory function is tracked largely by results of FVC. Patients should be informed about results of pulmonary function studies, prognosis, and palliative care options at each visit. The goal of patient education during palliation is to allow patients to make informed decisions about care. RCPs play a key role in educating patients and their families about the respiratory complications of ALS and the pros and cons of ventilation and secretion mobilization options. Most RCPs work with terminal illness in intensive care units and have experience in the final stages of respiratory disease. Specialized training in the management of chronic obstructive and restrictive lung disease, microprocessor mechanical ventilators, and artificial airways allow RCPs to answer the detailed questions patients and their families might have regarding respiratory support. Patient education is the foundation of informed consent, the patient's right to accept or refuse physician recommended therapies (Kaub-Wittemer et al., 2003).

The American Thoracic Society recommendations for patient education in Duchenne muscular dystrophy, another life-limited disease, are instructive. Successful education by the RCP will allow the patient to do the following:

- Understand the pulmonary progression of ALS and its clinical markers.
- Recognize signs and symptoms of pulmonary complications.
- Understand and make informed choices about treatment options for airway clearance and respiratory insufficiency. Education should include options for noninvasive ventilation as well as ventilation via tracheostomy. Risks, benefits, and QoL issues for the different ventilatory support options should be reviewed.
- Understand the role of respiratory medical devices in use and have sufficient skill to operate them effectively.
- Understand and make informed decisions about end-of-life care. Adapted from the American Thoracic Society Consensus Statement, Respiratory Care of the Patient with Duchenne Muscular Dystrophy, 2004.

After appropriate education has been provided, patient autonomy and self-determination in electing to accept or reject ventilatory support must be respected. RCPs should make every effort to keep biases and personal feelings about life support from influencing patients' choices.

Advanced Directives for Health Care

ADs are detailed descriptions of what kind of medical care a patient desires at the end-of-life. ADs allow patients to communicate their wishes to family members and medical staff if they are incapacitated and unable to do so themselves. Physicians and other healthcare personnel can assist the patient by explaining what life support measures entail (intubation, tracheostomy and mechanical ventilation, antibiotic therapy, nutritional support, hydration therapy), but the wording and decisions must be the patient's alone. Advances in life-sustaining measures have made decisions more complicated. Health care professionals can explain the options in layman's terms to assist the process. Disease-specific ADs have been advocated by physicians who treat patients with neuromuscular diseases as being more useful than broad, general statements (Benditt et al., 2001). Patients should be assured that they may change or revoke their AD at any time.

ADs can reduce anxiety and uncertainty at end-of-life because patients are assured family members will know their wishes for specific options, life support, or hospice care (Akabayashi et al., 2004). Many people think ADs are a good idea but believe they are not needed because family or physicians know their wishes (American Psychological Association, 2008). ADs alleviate the legal and ethical uncertainty for the physician that might lead to over treatment and "defensive medicine" (Akabayashi et al.). Discussion of end-of-life choices can promote trust among patients, family members, and clinicians.

ADs differ by state. Copies can be obtained from ALS clinics and hospitals, health departments, state departments on aging, and attorneys. A number of websites have versions that can be downloaded and printed, including the National Institute of Medicine. Recommended websites can be found in the Resources section.

Five Wishes is a document that helps patients express their personal, emotional, and spiritual needs, as well as medical wishes for how they want to be treated if they are unable to speak for themselves. It includes a proxy (also referred to as health care agent, representative, or surrogate) chosen to make decisions if the patient is unable to do so. Five Wishes can be purchased at www.agingwithdignity.org/5wishes.html. The document must be witnessed, signed, and notarized per state law.

Living wills, another type of AD, are written legal documents describing life-sustaining and medical treatments chosen or rejected at the end of life. Living wills do not allow the patient to choose a proxy.

A durable power of attorney (DPA) for health care is a legal document appointing a person to make medical decisions for a patient who becomes unable to do so. It is generally more useful than a living will. A DPA becomes active when the patient is unconscious or otherwise unable to communicate medical decisions. The DPA should be a trusted family member or friend who willingly accepts the responsibility and agrees to follow the patient's wishes.

Cultural Considerations

Culture determines a group's values and world view. Ethnicity is one's self-identified group and may include subgroups that share common values. Culture shapes decisions regarding resuscitation, mechanical ventilation, and feeding tubes. Healthcare professionals should respect patients' cultures and learn culturally competent strategies to explain illness and treatment options (American Psychological Association, 2008). A patient's culture may determine their attitude toward the following:

- Knowing of a terminal diagnosis
- Aggressiveness of care
- Dying at home
- Dying in a hospital, or a specific hospital
- Dying in hospice
- Being placed in a long-term care facility
- Tolerating pain and suffering

In the United States as a whole, individual autonomy is highly valued, but individual self-determination is valued less than family and community wishes within some minority cultures. Some Koreans expect the eldest son to make decisions for his parents at the end of life (American Psychological Association, 2008). Designated family decision makers in other immigrant cultures may be brothers, uncles, fathers, or other relatives who may live outside the United States and will need to be consulted.

Attitudes toward discussing death and how aggressively to intervene vary a great deal. Talking about death itself may be taboo. Some Koreans and Zuni believe that discussing death with a patient can hasten death. In the African American community, aggressive treatment is more commonly favored than among other groups. Latinos hold differing views, with one third opposing life support and most unfamiliar with hospice. Muslims believe that treatments that have become futile are not mandatory (American Psychological Association, 2008). In trying to educate ourselves about common traditions and tendencies of patients from a specific culture, however, we risk oversimplifying and generalizing the complex needs of individuals. The person behind the patient can be found by asking, checking, and listening to their wants and needs (Oliviere et al., 2004).

The first hospice in the United States was opened in 1974. Today there are 4500 hospices with the greatest growth in small, freestanding programs (National Palliative Care and Hospice Organizations, 2002). Nationally, hospices serve mostly whites (81%), and few Native Americans (0.3%), African Americans (8%), Asian, Hawaiian, and Pacific Islanders (1.8%), and Hispanics (3%). In California, only 32% of people who had lost a loved one in the past year knew "a lot" about hospice, although 71% "had heard of it." People who were older, white, and had higher economic levels reported more familiarity with hospice and were more likely to hold positive views of this program (California Healthcare Foundation, 2006).

In November 2006, the California Healthcare Foundation published the results of a statewide survey "Attitudes toward End-of-Life Care in California." The results of the survey focused attention on cultural differences and special concerns of racial minorities: language barriers, communication barriers between medical staff and family members, and finding staff that were sensitive to cultural differences. Two thirds of African Americans (65%) and 60% of Chinese Americans (Mandarin or Cantonese-speaking) were very concerned about "finding health care providers who (would) understand and respect their beliefs and values."

California is a large and culturally diverse state, sitting on the Pacific Rim and sharing a border with Mexico. The end-of-life survey conducted among members of major cultural and ethnic groups who had lost a loved one during the previous year is instructive (Tables 11-1–11-3).

Within the same culture, there are differences based on geography, gender, age, religion, socioeconomic status, and degree of cultural

Table 11-1 End-of-life choice with a terminal illness

Race/ethnicity	Wish to Die	Depends	Do Everything
White	69%	14%	14%
Latino	39%	14%	44%
African American	38%	14%	44%
Asian/non-Chinese	43%	23%	28%
Chinese*	34%	25%	39%

*Mandarin or Cantonese-speaking
California Healthcare Foundation End-of-Life Survey, November 2006

Table 11-2 Would want life support removed
if in a persistent coma

White	87%
Latino	70%
African American	72%
Asian/non-Chinese	83%
Chinese	79%

California Healthcare Foundation End-of-Life Survey,
November 2006

Table 11-3 The primary concerns of Californians at end-of-life based
on reported race

White	Pain and discomfort; being a burden to family and friends
Latino	Not being able to afford the care you need; being at peace spiritually
African-American	Finding providers who respect your culture; being at peace spiritually
Asian/non-Chinese	Not being able to afford the care you need; pain and discomfort
Chinese	Not being able to afford the care you need; being a burden to family and friends

California Healthcare Foundation End-of-Life Survey, November 2006

assimilation. The United States is rich in cultural diversity, and each patient will need to be approached in an individualized way. Being open to cultures different from one's own requires a close look at personal values, assumptions, biases, and end-of-life views. Recognizing one's own viewpoint and acknowledging the family, culture, and country from which it arose allow for a greater acceptance of views that are different. At the end of this chapter is a values history questionnaire that can assist in this process (Appendix 11-1).

No health care provider, no matter how well motivated, can become an expert on the end-of-life values of all other possible cultures they may encounter. The most important thing that we can do is recognize that we lack information we need to understand the values of a specific patient and do all we can to educate ourselves about them. Most families will be happy to answer questions about their value system if approached in an open, nonjudgmental manner.

RESPIRATORY FAILURE

Mechanical Ventilation

ALS entails an inevitable progression to respiratory failure. Patients are monitored closely, and patients' wishes are reviewed at each turning point. As ALS progresses, the goal of patient care changes from maximizing function to providing effective and compassionate palliative care (Miller, 2007).

The American Academy of Neurology practice parameter recommends the following:

1. Be vigilant for symptoms indicating hypoventilation. Serial measures of pulmonary function (especially vital capacity) are recommended to guide management and determine prognosis with the understanding that no single test can reliably detect hypoventilation. (Guideline)

2. Offer noninvasive ventilatory support as an effective initial therapy for symptomatic chronic hypoventilation and to prolong survival in patients with ALS. (Guideline)

3. When long-term survival is the goal, offer invasive ventilation and fully inform patient and family of burdens and benefits. (Guideline)

4. In accordance with the principle of patient autonomy, physicians should respect the right of the patient with ALS to refuse or withdraw any treatment, including mechanical ventilation. (Guideline)

5. When withdrawing ventilation, use adequate opiates and anxiolytics to relieve dyspnea and anxiety. (Guideline)

It is a strong consensus of both the ALS Task Force and the Quality Standards Subcommittee of the AAN that during withdrawal of ventilation, paralyzing drugs should not be used because patients may not be able to express pain or distress (Miller et al., 1999).

A loss of bulbar muscle tone and inability to clear secretions and risk of aspiration may limit the use of NPPV; therefore, patients with bulbar ALS may not tolerate NPPV, and invasive ventilation should be considered (Bach, 1995; Heffernan et al., 2006; Miller et al., 1999).

When a patient can no longer tolerate NPPV or NPPV is ineffective in providing sufficient ventilation and oxygenation, he or she must choose between tracheostomy and mechanical ventilation (life support) or hospice

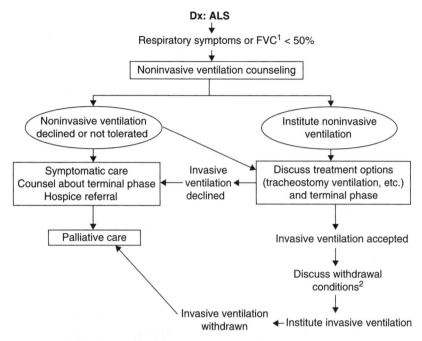

Dx: ALS

Respiratory symptoms or FVC[1] < 50%

Noninvasive ventilation counseling

Noninvasive ventilation declined or not tolerated

Institute noninvasive ventilation

Symptomatic care
Counsel about terminal phase
Hospice referral

Invasive ventilation declined

Discuss treatment options (tracheostomy ventilation, etc.) and terminal phase

Palliative care

Invasive ventilation accepted

Discuss withdrawal conditions[2]

Invasive ventilation withdrawn

Institute invasive ventilation

[1]FVC (forced vital capacity) or SVC (slow vital capacity) can be used; SVC may be more accurate in patients with bulbar dysfunction

[2]Agreement needed for conditions of withdrawal, prior to, or concurrent with, instituting invasive ventilation (e.g. locked-instate, coma, etc.)

FIGURE 11-1 Algorithm for Respiratory Management. Reprinted with permission from: Amyotrophic Lateral Sclerosis: American Academy of Neurology Press Quality of Life Guide Series. Robert G. Miller, MD, Deborah Gelinas, MD, Patricia O'Connor, RN © 2004, Demos Medical Publishing

care (Figure 11-1). The cost and possible benefit of mechanical ventilation (financial, social, and emotional for patient and caregivers) should be discussed (Heffernan et al., 2006; Miller 2007). Patients using mechanical ventilation may live months or years from time of tracheostomy; however, patients may progress to a "locked in" syndrome in which all muscles will be fully paralyzed. Death commonly occurs from pneumonia or cardiovascular disease.

Predictors of Elective Long-Term Mechanical Ventilation

The prevalence of long-term mechanical ventilation (LTMV) in ALS varies within and among countries. LTMV is influenced by insurance coverage (national or private) and resource allocation, physician attitudes, ethical and legal considerations, cultural standards (whether the physician, patient, or the family makes the decision), and as the result of unplanned emergency intubation and ventilation (Borasio et al., 1998; Rabkin et al., 2006; Smyth et al., 1997; Kaub-Wittemer et al. 2003).

An estimate of the number of elective tracheostomies in ALS in North America is 3% (Miller et al., 2000). In North America, and especially in the United States, medical care has a strong tradition of being patient driven (Borasio et al., 1998). Rabkin et al. (2006) sought to characterize ALS patients who opt for tracheostomy and LTMV. In a prospective study of 72 hospice eligible patients, patients who chose LTMV and those who declined and died were compared with respect to medical, psychiatric, and psychosocial measures. Factors contributing to elective LTMV were younger age, having young children, higher education, and higher household income on average than patients who refused life support. The strongest independent predictors of voluntary LTMV were patient age and having children under 21. Physical conditions were similar between the two groups. Patients who chose LTMV reported more positive appraisals of their ability to function in daily life, physical health, and overall well-being and life satisfaction. Those opting for LTMV had higher levels of optimism (including a belief that a cure was imminent), faith in the future, positive expectations, and enthusiasm. LTMV users were less likely to be clinically depressed and were more likely to be using antidepressant medication; however, depression was not a significant predictor of the decision to forego tracheostomy and ventilation. There was no clinically significant cognitive impairment among LTMV users. Religious beliefs and affiliation did not differ significantly between the two groups. Residence (home or institution) did not impact the decision to prolong life. Although not statistically significant, the LTMV group was more likely to have used NPPV continuously (24 hours per day) than those who chose not to prolong life.

LTMV was chosen not out of desperation, ignorance, or inability to communicate end-of-life wishes. Instead, the authors concluded this: "LTMV choice was consistent with a sustained sense that life was worth living in any way possible, at least for some time and within certain boundaries." These results are supported by other studies that conclude that ventilator-dependent patients with ALS are not more depressed than patients who are not ventilator dependent (MacDonald et al., 1996) and can lead meaningful lives (Moss et al., 1993, 1996). For patients who are sustained on mechanical ventilation, either by choice or as the result of acute respiratory failure, 90% of those cared for at home are satisfied with LTMV (Moss et al., 1993), as are 72% cared for in an institutional setting (Cazzolli & Oppenheimer, 1996).

Medical personnel may judge incorrectly that patients would be dissatisfied with life on a ventilator (Bach et al., 1991). One cannot judge another's QoL. If a patient has chosen to be supported through invasive mechanical ventilation, the RCP should assist with the transition through coordination with durable medical equipment providers, caregiver education and training, and ongoing support.

Withdrawal of Life Support

Patients with ALS who are mechanically ventilated by choice or after unplanned, emergency intubation may choose to have life support withdrawn. In the 1970s and 1980s, the act of withdrawing life support treatment was considered "passive euthanasia" because death was considered to be the result of the discontinuation of life support. Today, death that results from withholding or discontinuing life support is seen as the natural outcome of a terminal disease (Bernat, 2004). Legal and ethical precedents support the right of a mentally competent, informed patient to discontinue life support and mechanical ventilation, and healthcare providers are required to respect such as request (Miller et al., 1999).

Terminal Stage

Proper palliative care is essential when respiratory failure will result from a patient's decision to withdraw or refuse noninvasive positive pressure ventilation or invasive mechanical ventilation. Palliative care can take place at home, hospital, or long-term care facility. Patients and loved ones should be assured that over 90% of patients with ALS die peacefully as increasing hypercapnia leads to drowsiness, sleep, and finally coma (Neudert et al., 2001). The primary cause of death (86%) is respiratory failure, followed by heart failure (6%) and pneumonia (5%). In the terminal stage, there is usually a gradual deterioration and then a sudden change over hours or a few days; 48% to 72% of patients deteriorate and die within 24 hours (Oliver & Borasio, 2004).

Symptom Control

Breath is life. Dyspnea at the end of life creates anxiety and dread at impending death. Patients and family members should be reassured that symptoms will be effectively controlled. The steps to managing symptoms of dyspnea, pain, and anxiety during withdrawal of mechanical ventilation on critical care units form the basis of the humane procedures carried out in the home and non-tertiary care centers (Wilson et al., 1992).

Dyspnea

Oral and Parenteral Treatment

Opioids are the treatment of choice for shortness of breath at the end of life; 81% of hospice patients with ALS found opioids to successfully relieve dyspnea (O'Brien et al., 1992). Low-dose morphine (5 mg) reduces dyspnea without causing respiratory depression (Borasio & Kaub-Wittemer, 2004). Family members may fear that administration of morphine by mouth or parenterally is active euthanasia. They should be assured that relief of discomfort is the primary goal of opioid administration. Respiratory depression may be a secondary effect, especially in older patients, but is an unintended consequence of symptom management.

Effective treatment for dyspnea includes initial 2.5- to 5.0-mg administration of morphine subcutaneously or transdermally or oral equivalent by mouth in the opioid-naïve patient every 4 hours and titrating upward as needed. Patients already receiving opioids for pain will need a starting dose 25% to 50% higher. For acute dyspnea, an increase of 1.5 mg every 10 minutes may be required. For severe dyspnea, continuous intravenous morphine infusion is recommended. Controlled-release morphine is often less effective for dyspnea treatment (Borasio & Kaub-Wittemer, 2004; Miller et al., 1999).

Aerosolized Treatments for Dyspnea

There are no controlled studies of aerosolized opioids in ALS. In uncontrolled studies and case reports, aerosolized opioids have been shown to relieve dyspnea better than parenteral opioids with fewer systemic adverse effects (nausea, constipation) in patients with terminal lung cancer and cystic fibrosis (Kallet, 2007). Other studies have found no benefit of aerosolized opioids, especially in advanced disease (Noseda et al., 1997).

Signs of sedation or respiratory depression were not observed in the majority of studies on inhaled opioids. If aerosolized opioids find their way into the gastrointestinal tract (due to oropharyngeal impaction of aerosol particles and subsequent swallowing), hypercapnia and respiratory depression can occur (Lang & Jedeikin, 1998).

The medulla is rich in opiate receptors, and peripheral opioid receptors occur throughout the body, which may explain the role of exogenous opiates on respiratory drive (Kallet, 2007). It has been hypothesized that pulmonary receptors (C-fiber irritant receptors in the central and peripheral airways, J-receptors, and stretch receptors in the alveolar walls) may respond to inhaled opiates. If opiates can modulate the discrepancy that occurs between effort (signals from the cortex) and force (inspiratory muscles) and displacement (lung and chest wall) that occurs in end-stage restrictive lung disease, resulting dyspnea can be controlled (Kallet, 2007).

In small, generally uncontrolled studies, aerosolized furosemide (Lasix) has been shown to relieve dyspnea in patients with terminal cancer (Shimoyama & Shimoyama, 2002). Delivering furosemide through nebulization is thought to control dyspnea by decreasing the respiratory rate and use of accessory muscles. It is hypothesized that inhaled furosemide is able to stimulate pulmonary stretch receptors by mimicking large tidal volumes (Kallet, 2007).

Oxygen

The role of oxygen at the end of life is controversial in ALS. It has been a mainstay of palliative and hospice care in the treatment of dyspnea, although its benefit has not been documented. It should be used to treat documented hypoxia. In ALS, respiratory compromise is due to respiratory muscle weakness and not airway or alveolar impairment. Chronic hypercapnia is common in late stage ALS. Oxygen administration may lead to hypoventilation, somnolence, and respiratory arrest (Borasio & Kaub-Wittemer, 2004).

Anxiety

Although well-controlled studies do not exist, anxiolytics are frequently used to manage dyspnea at the end of life. Anxiety and fear can accompany or result in dyspnea. Lorazepam administered sublingually (0.5 to 2.5 mg) or diazepam rectally (2.5 to 5.0 mg) are effective (Borasio &

Kaub-Wittemer, 2004). For terminal restlessness and confusion caused by hypercapnia, a neuroleptic such as chlorpromazine (Thorazine) 25 mg every 4 to 12 hours rectally or 12.5 mg every 4 to 12 hours by mouth, intravenously, or parenterally is recommended (Andersen et al., 2005; Miller et al., 1999).

Pain

Pain is relatively common in the later stages of ALS because of stiff joints from immobility and muscle cramps. Antispasticity, anti-inflammatory, and analgesic medications have been used successfully (Miller et al., 1999). Antidepressants (amitriptyline or selective serotonin reuptake inhibitors) can assist with pain management during the course of ALS. When nonnarcotics fail, opioids have been reported to alleviate pain in 80% of ALS patients at the end of life (Miller et al., 1999).

Nonpharmacological Treatments

Alternative and complementary treatments may be useful in managing symptoms of dyspnea. Acupuncture has been studied in the relief of breathlessness. Relaxation techniques, breathing retaining, and guided imagery may be helpful (Krishnasamy et al., 2001). A fan or fresh air flowing toward the patient may be helpful. This is possibly due to the stimulation of mechanoreceptors on the face (Borasio & Kaub-Wittemer, 2004). A calm environment, favorite music, loved pets, distractions (being read to), and proximity of loved ones may be important methods of palliation.

Psychosocial Factors

ALS has a negative impact on the QoL of patients and their caregivers (Lo Coco et al., 2005). There are only mild-to-moderate correlations between psychological and physical health symptoms. Patients who may report good QoL, despite declines in functioning, point to the role of health perception in overall outlook. Maintaining a good QoL is affected by the successful treatment of distressing symptoms (respiratory insufficiency, sialorrhea, pseudobulbar affect), living situation, and economic well-being. Social relationships and family relationships are essential (Rabkin et al., 2006).

Spouses and partners of people with ALS have reported that their QoL was reduced when tracheostomy and ventilation are chosen. Finding and affording qualified assistance in the home is difficult (Rabkin et al., 2006). Caregivers of patients on LTMV have reported being heavily burdened and outside activities severely limited (Gelinas et al., 1998). The emotional burdens are great, but caregivers also report a great deal of satisfaction in their role (Rabkin et al.). Caregivers who report lower QoL levels are not always those who have to look after the most physically or psychologically impaired patients (Lo Coco et al., 2005). Patients may underestimate the burdens imposed by their decision to prolong life through ventilatory support (Rabkin et al.).

Publication of *The 36-Hour Day* in 1981 introduced the general public to the crucial role of family and friends in caring for seriously ill loved ones and the need for services, respite care, and support (Mace & Rabins, 1981). The monetary value of services provided by informal caregivers is estimated at $306 billion annually (Family Caregiver Alliance, 2008). Today, local, national, and international organizations for people with ALS and their caregivers provide emotional and practical support, information, and advocacy. Support organizations are listed in the resource section.

Depression can occur when there is a large gap between a person's expectations of life and the reality they face. Sadness on learning of an ALS diagnosis is appropriate. A depressed mood that lasts for weeks, especially if it is accompanied by feelings of hopelessness, lack of motivation, sleep disturbances, and loss of appetite should be evaluated. Cognitive therapy has been shown to be effective. Antidepressants can be considered.

Wish to Die and Hastened Death

Documented suicide among ALS patients is low (Neudert et al., 2001; Oliver & Borasio, 2004). In the United States, many patients with amyotrophic lateral sclerosis show an interest in physician-assisted suicide (Grazini et al., 1998). In a prospective study of 80 patients with late-stage ALS, of the 53 who died during the course of the study, 10 (18.9%) had expressed the wish to die (chose not to accept life-prolonging measures), and 3 (5.7%) ended their own lives. Patients who expressed a wish to die were less optimistic, found less comfort in religion, and felt greater hopelessness but did not rate significantly higher on depression scales than those who wanted to continue to live. Patients wishing to die were clear that death would be preferable to suffering and disability at the end of life. Patients who expressed a wish to die did not avail themselves of life-prolonging treatments like noninvasive positive pressure ventilation and were less likely to accept feeding tubes.

Patients who ended their lives reported reduction in suffering and increased perception of control over ALS in the final weeks of life. Depression was less severe in the patients who ended their lives than those who expressed a wish to die but did not act on it. Patients who ultimately took their own lives began with the highest ratings of suffering, based on self-rated states listed on a visual analogue scale. Suffering declined as the time to death approached. Suffering increased in patients who did not act on the wish to die and in the patients who did not express a wish to die (Albert et al., 2005). In Oregon, the only state in which physician-assisted suicide is legal, patients who have been granted the permission and means to hasten death with physician assistance have also reported a sense of increased control. Patients must submit a written request for physician assistance in hastening death on two separate occasions and have depression ruled out as a factor in making the request.

Albert et al. (2005) raise a number of questions of interest to medical personnel who work with life-limiting diseases:

- Can depression in end-stage disease be separated from existential suffering, a more general loss of meaning and purpose?
- Is the desire to hasten death a feature of depression or of a broader syndrome of "end-of-life despair" (suffering, loss of interest in living, absence of pleasure, loss of interest in activity, and pessimism)?
- Can the ability to control existential suffering through the option of hastened death be considered an element of dignity at the end of life?

RCP ATTITUDES TOWARD TERMINATING LIFE SUPPORT

There are no published studies of RCPs in palliative and end-of-life care (Giordano, 2000); however, RCPs routinely participate in the termination of life support in their role of managing mechanical ventilation in intensive care units (Rubenfeld, 2000). To assess attitudes and concerns of RCPs regarding withdrawing life support measures, Willms and Brewer (2005) conducted a survey of 119 RCPs working in acute-care hospitals in a large, urban area. Ninety-six percent of respondents had conducted terminal extubation as part of their clinical responsibilities. Respondents had an average of 14.5 years of practice (range, 1 to 35 years) and on average had been involved in terminal extubation 33 times in the course of their career. Physicians were at the bedside in only a small minority of these extubations; however, RCPs were generally not included in the multidisciplinary team conferences, at which terminal extubation was decided.

Willms and Brewer (2005) asked survey participants to rank three roles of RCPs in order of greatest importance. RCPs ranked ensuring QoL highest (29.4%), followed by relieving suffering (27.7%) and preserving life (24.4%), with 18.5% not being sure. Respondents desired a role in the end-of-life decision-making process and more definitive physician orders for terminal extubation. Only 45% of RCPs had received education on end-of-life care or termination of life support in respiratory therapy programs and 33% during hospital-based continuing education programs. A majority of respondents expressed a desire for education regarding terminal care. Rubenfeld (2000) agreed, stating that withdrawal of life support should be treated like any other medical procedure with proper planning, education, documentation, and quality-improvement initiatives.

RESPIRATORY CONTROVERSIES AT END OF LIFE

The Role of NPPV at the End of Life

Evidence-based reviews of the management of symptoms in ALS include NPPV as a way to alleviate hypoventilation and dyspnea and improve QoL (Andersen et al., 2005; Heffernan et al., 2006; Miller et al., 1999). Noninvasive ventilation decreases mortality in the short run but will be unable to sustain life as the disease progresses. There is disagreement among hospice practitioners and RCPs about whether NPPV is a component of palliative care or a life-prolonging measure.

RT Magazine published a point/counterpoint discussion in which RCPs Nuccio and Whitnack debated the role of NPPV at the end of life. Although ALS was not specifically addressed, discussion of NPPV use in end-stage cancer, cystic fibrosis, and chronic obstructive pulmonary disease is relevant to RCPs working with patients with neuromuscular disease as these diseases share symptoms of respiratory insufficiency.

NPPV for Palliation

Nuccio (2006) argued that NPPV allows flexibility at the end of life. He described it as an important adjunct to palliative care as it reduces the work of breathing by improving alveolar ventilation and reducing hypercapnia and hypoxia. Air hunger is one of the most distressing symptoms of hypoventilation, both for the patient and the loved ones caring for them. By reducing dyspnea, the use of NPPV can allow patients to avoid or reduce the use of narcotics and anxiolytics and the accompanying side effects of somnolence and constipation. For patients who refuse terminal sedation on the grounds that they want to be fully present with their loved ones at the end of life, NPPV may serve as an option for managing shortness of breath.

For patients who arrive in the emergency department in acute respiratory failure without an AD but who remain ambivalent about intubation and mechanical ventilation, NPPV can be used to manage symptoms and provide patient and family with time for discussion of end-of-life options. Nuccio (2006) suggested NPPV be included as one of the comfort care options in addition to oxygen and pharmacological agents and encouraged the American College of Chest Physicians to expand and clarify their position statement on the issue.

NPPV as Prolongation of Life

Whitnack (2006) states this: "When patients opt for comfort care, that is what we should offer them, not an artificial prolongation of life." He speaks specifically of the patient who has a written "do not resuscitate/do not intubate" directive. Whitnack sees NPPV use in patients with DNR/DNI orders as symptomatic of the lack of end-of-life training of many physicians and reflective of a denial of death. He sees NPPV use as collusion between medical staff and patients in not fully facing the last moments of life and fostering the illusion that death is not imminent.

Whitnack (2006) views NPPV as a life prolonging measure. Removal of the mask then becomes a method of hastening death instead of death resulting from natural causes. Low-dose morphine has been shown to be successful in managing dyspnea without causing drowsiness, and therefore, NPPV is unnecessary to manage symptoms of hypoventilation.

Whitnack sites his own palliative care unit in which physicians trained to manage end-of-life symptoms did not prescribe NPPV. It also appears that indeed NPPV can prolong life in the event of an exacerbation of underlying pulmonary disease. If physicians intervene to treat an acute respiratory event, Whitnack argues, the patient will certainly face another exacerbation in the future, prolonging the inevitable. Whitnack asks in this case "whether we are helping to prolong the living process or prolong the dying process."

Discontinuance of NPPV: Who, When, Where, Why, and How

No matter why NPPV was initiated, at the end of life, its withdrawal must be considered a step-wise process and approached deliberately with all of those affected (patient, loved ones, and staff) (Johnson, 2007). When discontinuation of NPPV will result in progression to death of a conscious patient, his or her intent must be ascertained. Withdrawal can be begun when

- A predetermined endpoint has been reached, as specified in the patient's AD
- The patient or proxy requests it
- When the limits of NPPV to adequately ventilate the patient have been reached
- In an unresponsive patient, when loved ones perceive unacceptable levels of pain or suffering have been reached

NPPV should be discontinued in a setting where the patient, friends, and family are most comfortable (home, inpatient unit with palliative care service, or hospice). The location should be one where health care professionals are comfortable administering care at the end of life. The end of life should come where there are sufficient family, friends, and medical staff to provide care of the patient and emotional support of the family.

Withdrawal of NPPV (removal of mask) should be accompanied by premedication with opiates and anxiolytics, with doses titrated incrementally as needed to relieve dyspnea and anxiety. The patient should be monitored for signs of discomfort and efforts made to alleviate it. Family and friends should be told that time to death after NPPV has been discontinued is variable and that opiates and anxiolytics may prolong rather than hasten dying (Edwards, 2005).

SUMMARY

When there is no cure for a disease, the emphasis becomes comfort and caring. Caring for people with ALS is multidimensional. It allows RCPs to meld knowledge of respiratory assessment and symptom management with the other aspects of a patient's life: social, psychological, spiritual, and existential. RCPs spend the bulk of time focused on medical issues. At the end of life, nonmedical issues become important: having relationships with friends and family, savoring past pleasures, yearning for lost opportunities, and contemplating the meaning of life. Exploring these issues becomes part of the healing process.

RCPs are providers of palliative care in ALS because of their knowledge of restrictive lung disease. Knowledge of advancements in portable invasive and noninvasive ventilators allows RCPs to recommend options for home care and mobility. Opportunities exist for research into and development of best practice models for lung hyperinflation and secretion mobilization therapies at this level of care.

RCPs can play a significant role in making an inevitable death a good one, one that the patient and their loved ones want. At the end of life, patients want to know their options for ventilation and ways to minimize respiratory discomfort. Patients need assurance that health care professionals will be a resource and support them until the end. It is a great comfort to know that every effort will be made to relieve suffering and value life until the last breath is taken.

REFERENCES

Akabayashi A, Slingsby BT, Voltz R. Advance directives. In Voltz R, Bernat JL, Borasio GD, et al. (eds.). *Palliative Care in Neurology*. New York: Oxford University Press; 2004.

Albert SM, Murphy PL, Del Bene ML, Rowland LP. A prospective study of preferences and actual treatment choices in ALS. *Neurology* 1999;53: 278–282.

Albert SM, Rabkin JG, Del Bene ML, et al. Wish to die in end-stage ALS. *Neurology* 2005;65:68–74.

American Psychological Association Ad Hoc Committee on End of Life Issues. Culturally diverse communication and end-of-life care. Available at www.apa. org/pi/eol/fsculturallydiverse. Accessed July 1, 2008.

American Thoracic Society Consensus Statement. Respiratory care of the patient with Duchenne muscular dystrophy. *Am J Respir Crit Care Med* 2004;170:456–465. Available at www.atsjournals.org.

Andersen PM, Borasio GD, Dengler R, et al. EFNS task force on management of amyotrophic lateral sclerosis: guidelines for diagnosing and clinical care of patients and relatives: an evidence-based review with good practice points. *Eur J Neurol* 2005;12:921–938.

Bach JR. Amyotrophic lateral sclerosis: predictors for prolongation of life by noninvasive respiratory aids. *Arch Phys Med Rehab* 1995;76:828–832.

Bach JR, Campagnolo DI, Hoeman S. Life satisfaction of individuals with Duchenne muscular dystrophy using long-term mechanical ventilatory support. *Am J Phys Med Rehab* 1991;70:129–135.

Benditt JO, Smith TS, Tonelli MR. Empowering the individual with ALS at end-of-life: disease specific advance care planning. *Muscle Nerve* 2001;24:1706–1709.

Bernat JL. Refusal and withdrawal of treatment. In Voltz R, Bernat JL, Borasio GD, et al. (eds.). *Palliative Care in Neurology.* New York: Oxford University Press; 2004.

Borasio GD, Gelinas DF, Yanagisawa N. Mechanical ventilation in amyotrophic lateral sclerosis: a cross-cultural perspective. *J Neurol* 1998m245(Suppl 2): S7–S12.

Borasio GD, Kaub-Wittemer D. Respiratory symptoms. In Voltz R, Bernat JL, Borasio GD, et al. (eds.). *Palliative Care in Neurology.* New York: Oxford University Press; 2004.

California Healthcare Foundation. Attitudes toward end-of-life care in California. November 2006. Available at www.chcf.org/documents/chronicdisease/ EOLsurvey. Accessed July 2, 2008.

Cazzolli PA, Oppenheimer EA. Home mechanical ventilation for amyotrophic lateral sclerosis: nasal compared to tracheostomy-intermittent positive pressure ventilation. *J Neurol Sci* 1996;139:123–128.

Christakis NA. Death foretold: prophecy and prognosis in medical care. Chicago: University of Chicago Press; 1999.

Edwards M. Opioids and benzodiazepines appear paradoxically to delay inevitable death after ventilation withdrawal. *J Palliat Care* 2005;21:299–302.

Family Caregiver Alliance. Available at www.caregiver.org/caregiver/jsp/content_ node.jsp?nodeid=566. Accessed July 2, 2008.

Gelinas DF, O'Connor P, Miller RG. Quality of life for ventilator-dependent patients and their caregivers. *J Neurol Sci* 1998;160(Suppl 1): S134–S136.

Giordano M. The respiratory therapist and palliative care. *Respir Care* 2000;45: 1468–1474.

Grazini L, Johnson WS, McFarland BH, et al. Attitudes of patients with amyotrophic lateral sclerosis and their caregivers toward assisted suicide. *N Engl J Med* 1998;339:967–973.

Heffernan C, Jenkinson C, Holmes T, et al. Management of respiration in MND/ALS patients: an evidence based review. *Amyotrophic Lateral Sclerosis* 2006;7: 5–15.

Johnson W. Withdrawal of respiratory care: end of life issues. Presented at the Amyotrophic Lateral Sclerosis Association Will Rogers Institute Respiratory Symposium. January 27–28, 2007.

Kallet RH. The role of inhaled opiods and furosemide for the treatment of dyspnea. *Respir Care* 2007;52:901–910.

Kaub-Wittemer D, von Steinbuchel, Wasner M. Quality of life and psychosocial issue in ventilated patients with amyotrophic lateral sclerosis and their caregivers. *J Pain Symptom Manage* 2003;26:890–896.

Krishnasamy M, Corner J, Bredin M. Cancer nursing practice development: understanding breathlessness. *J Clin Nurs* 2001;10:103–108.

Lang E, Jedeikin R. Acute respiratory depression as a complication of nebulized morphine. *Can J Ansesth* 1998;45:60–62.

Lo Coco, G, Lo Coco D, Cicero V, et al. Individual and health-related quality of life assessment in amyotrophic lateral sclerosis patients and their caregivers. *J Neurol Sci* 2005;238:11–17.

MacDonald ER, Hillel A, Wiedenfeld SA. Evaluation of the psychological status of ventilator-supported patients with ALS/MND. *Palliat Med* 1996;10:35–41.

Mace NL, Rabins PV. *The 36-Hour Day: A Family Guide to Caring for Persons With Alzheimer's Disease, Related Dementing Illnes, and Memory Loss in Later Life.* Baltimore, MD: The Johns Hopkins University Press; 1981.

Maddocks I. Palliative care education for neurologists. In Voltz R, Bernat JL, Borasio GD, et al. (eds.). *Palliative Care in Neurology.* New York: Oxford University Press; 2004.

Miller RG. Treatment for respiratory insufficiency in ALS: evidence based management. Presented at the Amyotrophic Lateral Sclerosis Association Will Rogers Institute Respiratory Symposium, Newport Beach, CA. January 27, 2007.

Miller RG, Rosenberg JA, Gelinas DF, et al. Practice parameter: the care of the patient with amyotrophic lateral sclerosis (an evidence-based review): report of the Quality Standards Committee of the American Academy of Neurology: ALS Practice Parameters Task Force. *Neurology* 1999;52:1311–1323.

Miller RG, Anderson F, Bradley W, et al. (the ALS CARE study group). The ALS CARE Program—North American Patient CARE database: goals, design, and early results. *Neurology* 2000;54:53-57.

Moss AH, Casey P, Stocking CB, et al. Home ventilation for amyotrophic lateral sclerosis patients: outcomes, costs, and patient, family, and physician attitudes. *Neurology* 1993;43:438–443.

Moss AH, Oppenheimer EA, Casey P, et al. Patients with amyotrophic lateral sclerosis receiving long-term mechanical ventilation: advance care planning and outcomes. *Chest* 1996;110:249–255.

Munroe CA, Sirdofsky MD, Kuru T, Anderson ED. End-of-life decision making in 42 patients with amyotrophic lateral sclerosis. *Respir Care* 2007;52:996–999.

National Palliative Care and Hospice Organizations. Hospice statistics and research, November 8, 2002. Available at www.lastacts.org. Funded by the Robert Wood Johnson Foundation. Accessed July 2, 2008.

Neudert C, Oliver D, Wasner M, Borasio GD. The course of the terminal phase in patients with amyotrophic lateral sclerosis. *J Neurol* 2001;248:612–616.

Noseda A, Carpiaux JP, Markstein C, et al. Disabling dyspnea in patients with advanced disease: lack of effect of nebulized morphine. *Eur Respir J* 1997;10:1079–1083.

Nuccio PF. NPPV is an important adjunct to palliative care. *RT Magazine*, August 2006. Available at www.rtmagazine.com/issues/articles/2006-08_02.asp. Accessed February 25, 2008.

O'Brien T, Kelly M, Saunders C. Motor neuron disease: a hospice perspective. *Br Med J* 1992;304:471–473.

Oliver D, Borasio GD. Diseases of motor nerves. In Voltz R, Bernat JL, Borasio GD, et al. (eds.). *Palliative Care in Neurology*. New York: Oxford University Press; 2004.

Oliviere D, Oliver D. Cultural aspects of care. In Voltz R, Bernat JL, Borasio GD, et al. (eds.). *Palliative Care in Neurology*. New York: Oxford University Press; 2004.

Rabkin JG, Albert AM, Tider T, et al. Predictors and course of elective long-term mechanical ventilation: a prospective study of ALS patients. *Amyotrophic Lateral Sclerosis* 2006;7:86–95.

Respiratory Care: Journal of the American Association for Respiratory Care. Conference on palliative respiratory care. *Respir Care* 2000;45 November and December.

Rubenfeld GD. Withdrawing life-sustaining treatment in the intensive care unit. *Respir Care* 2000;45:1399–1407.

Shimoyama N, Shimoyama M. Nebulized furosemide as a novel treatment for dyspnea in terminal cancer patients. *J Pain Symptom Manage* 2002;23:73–76.

Silverstein MD, Stocking CB, Antel JP, et al. Amyotrophic lateral sclerosis and life-sustaining therapy: patients' desires for information, participation in decision making, and life-sustaining therapy. *Mayo Clin Proc* 1991;66:906–913.

Smyth A, Riedl M, Kimura R, et al. End of life decisions in amyotrophic lateral sclerosis: a cross-cultural perspective. *J Neurol Sci* 1997;152(Suppl 1):S93–S96.

Voltz R, Borasio G. Palliative therapy in the terminal stage of neurological disease. *Neurology* 1997;244(Suppl 4):S2–S10.

Weeks JC, Cook EF, O'Day SJ, et al. Relationship between cancer patients' predictions of prognosis and their treatment preferences. *JAMA* 1998;279:1709–1714.

Whitnack J. NPPV does not have a positive role to play in the care of DRR/DNI. *RT Magazine*, August 2006. Available at www.rtmagazine.com/issues/articles/2006-08_02.asp. Accessed February 25, 2008.

Willms DC, Brewer JA. Survey of respiratory therapists' attitudes and concerns regarding terminal extubation. *Respir Care* 2005;50:1046.

Wilson WA, Smedira NG, Fink C, et al. Ordering and administration of sedatives and analgesics during the withholding and withdrawal of life support from critically ill patients. *JAMA* 1992;267:949–953.

World Health Organization. 2002. World Health Organization Definition of Palliative Care. Available at www.who.int/cancer/main.cfm. Accessed June 30, 2008.

Appendix 11-1

A Values History Questionnaire

1. What do you value most about your life (e.g., living a long life, living an active life, enjoying the company of family and friends)?

2. How do you feel about death and dying? Do you fear death and dying? Have you experienced the loss of a loved one? Did that person's illness or medical treatment influence your thinking about death and dying?

3. Do you believe life should always be preserved as long as possible?

4. If not, what kinds of mental or physical conditions would make you think that life-prolonging treatment should no longer be used?
   - Unaware of my life and surroundings
   - Unable to appreciate and continue the important relationships in my life
   - Unable to think well enough to make everyday decisions
   - In severe pain or discomfort

5. Could you imagine reasons for temporarily accepting medical treatment for the conditions that you described?

6. How much pain and risk would you be willing to accept if your chances of recovery from an illness or an injury were good (50/50 or better)?

7. What if your chances were poor (less than 1 in 10)?

8. Would your approach to accepting or rejecting care depend on how old you were at the time of treatment? Why?

9. Do you hold any religious or moral views about medicine or particular medical treatment?

10. Should financial considerations influence decisions about your medical care?

11. What other beliefs or values do you hold that should be considered by those making medical care decisions for you if you become unable to speak for yourself?

12. Most people have heard of difficult end-of-life situations involving family members or neighbors or people in the news. Have you had any reactions to those situations?

Adapted from the Vermont Ethics Network (www.vtethicsnetwork. org).

Resources

PROFESSIONAL ASSOCIATIONS FOR RESPIRATORY CARE PRACTITIONERS

American Association for Respiratory Care
http://www.aarc.org

The American Association for Respiratory Care (AARC) is a professional membership organization for respiratory care professionals and allied health specialists interested in cardiopulmonary care. The AARC publishes *AARC Times* and the peer-reviewed journal *Respiratory Care* and hosts the International Conference for Respiratory Care each December. The AARC focuses on patient and professional education, research, and public policy advocacy for patients and RCPs. Specialty sections include the following: continuing care/rehabilitation, diagnostics, home care, long-term care and sleep medicine. Members may elect to join the Neuromuscular Roundtable, an online discussion group of professionals working with patients with ALS and other neuromuscular diseases.

E-mail: neuro@AARC.org

The AARC site includes *Your Lung Health* for patients and family members.

The Association for Respiratory Technicians and Physiologists
http://www.artp.org.uk

The ARTP, along with the British Thoracic Society, provides national, professionally recognized competence qualifications in respiratory function testing and spirometry. The ARTP hosts an annual conference and publishes the journal *Inspire* three times a year.

241

The Canadian Society of Respiratory Therapists
http://www.csrt.com

The national professional association for respiratory therapists, the Canadian Society of Respiratory Therapists (CSRT) publishes the *Canadian Journal of Respiratory Therapy*; represents the profession on medical, government, education and advisory bodies; maintains a national professional standard of practice; works with health organizations concerned with asthma, emphysema, smoking, and health care; and awards the internationally recognized RRT credential.

International Council for Respiratory Care
http://www.irccouncil.org

The International Council for Respiratory Care (ICRC) is dedicated to advancing safe, effective and ethical practice of respiratory care through promoting the art, science, clinical practice and educational foundation required for the attainment of high quality respiratory care outcomes in all nations; developing and disseminating evidence-based standards of care according to the special needs and resources of individual nations; facilitating interaction among and between the allied health professions, nursing, the medical specialties, hospitals and clinics, service companies, and industry; encouraging the creation and growth of related respiratory care organizations in individual nations, and providing educational resources for patients, caregivers and the general public in respiratory health promotion, disease prevention, and rehabilitation as appropriate in individual nations.

The 1st International Respiratory Care Conference, hosted by Tawam Hospital, Al Ain, United Arab Emirates in affiliation with Johns Hopkins Medicine, was held in October 2008.

ORGANIZATIONS FOR PEOPLE WITH ALS, THEIR FAMILIES, AND MEDICAL PROFESSIONALS

ALS Association
http://www.alsa.org

The ALS Association is a not-for-profit voluntary health agency dedicated to the fight against ALS. Founded in 1985, over the past decade, ALSA has contributed over $40 million directly to research. Its Clinical Management Research Program focuses on the management of respiration, nutrition, mobility, and psychosocial needs of people with ALS. The Will Rogers Institute of the ALS Association funds research projects concerning clinical management of respiratory disease in ALS. ALSA supports a nationwide network of chapters that provide comprehensive services and support to ALS patients and families. It supports multidisciplinary clinics serving ALS patients. ALSA publishes patient education materials and caregiver resources and seeks to increase awareness of ALS and influence public policy through education and advocacy. It publishes a series of six booklets for patients and families *Living with ALS* that includes *Adapting to Breathing Changes*.

Muscular Dystrophy Association/ALS division
http://als.mdausa.org

MDA is a voluntary health agency that funds ALS research and direct services to people with ALS. The ALS division of the Muscular Dystrophy Association provides patient education and support groups for families and financial support for multidisciplinary clinics serving ALS patients. The MDA's 200 local offices maintain equipment loan closets and provide financial assistance for purchase and repair of wheelchairs, leg braces, and communication devices. It publishes *Quest*, a bimonthly news magazine, information booklets and pamphlets, and the comprehensive *Everyday Life with ALS: A Practical Guide*, free to families of those with ALS. Publications also include *When a Loved One Has ALS: A Caregiver's Guide* and *Breathe Easy: A Respiratory Guide for People Living with Neuromuscular Diseases*. E-mail: publications@mdausa.org.

Motor Neurone Disease Association
http://www.mndassociation.org

The Motor Neurone Disease Association is a resource for people with motor neuron disease and for those who care for them. The MND Association campaigns nationally and locally for better care for all people with MND and raises awareness of the disease. It hosts the annual International Symposium on ALS/MND, which brings together neurologists, pulmonologists, clinical practitioners, and allied health professionals who share the latest research and practice in MND/ALS.

Its mission is to fund and promote research to bring about an end to MND. Formed in 1979 by a group of volunteers, the MND Association now has 1500 volunteers and 120+ paid staff. It supports 15 multidisciplinary care centers across England, Wales, and Northern Ireland.

> Motor Neurone Disease Association. Guidelines. Northampton, UK: MNDA, 2006. Available at http://mndassociation.org/for_professionals/developing_services/guidelines.html.

RESOURCES FOR PEOPLE WITH ALS

Patients Like Me
http://www.patientslikeme.com/als/community

Patients Like Me is an online community for patients, caregivers, researchers, physicians, and allied health professionals in ALS care. People with ALS share their symptoms, treatments, treatment outcomes, and personal experiences to help themselves and others. The site has expanded and now includes specialty sections for HIV, MS, Parkinson's disease, and mood disorders.

International Ventilators Users Network
An affiliate of Post-Polio Health International
http://www.post-polio.org/ivun
E-mail: ventinfo@post-polio.org

The mission of the International Ventilator Users Network (IVUN) is to enhance the lives and independence of home mechanical ventilator users through education, advocacy, and networking. IVUN publishes the quarterly newsletter *Ventilator-Assisted Living* and hosts the International Home Ventilator Conference.

RESPIRATORY ASSISTIVE DEVICES AND SUPPLIES

CPAP.com (The CPAP store)
http://cpap.com

CPAP.com, formerly CPAPman.com, is an online store for the purchase of CPAP, bilevel positive pressure ventilation devices, masks, and other supplies. The site hosts CPAP talk, an online CPAP user's community, a newsletter, and a forum through which patients and clinicians can pose questions regarding sleep and adjusting to nocturnal positive airway pressure. The "CPAP man" is available to answer mask fitting and other adjustment and acclimation questions.

There are many online sites through which to purchase respiratory equipment and disposable supplies. Patients need a physician's prescription to purchase medical equipment. Clinical support after purchase is usually not available.

ADVANCED DIRECTIVES

Phillips LH II. Individual health care directive for the individual with amyotrophic lateral sclerosis. *J Clin Neuromusc Dis* 2002;3:116–121.

The American Academy of Family Physicians
Generic, downloadable advanced directive with explanations and definitions
http://www.aafp.org/afp/990201ap/617.html

Aging with Dignity
www.agingwithdignity.org/5wishes/html

Aging with Dignity sells the popular advanced directive *The Five Wishes.*

The *Five Wishes* document helps you express how you want to be treated if you are seriously ill and unable to speak for yourself. It is unique among all other living will and health agent forms because it looks to all of a person's needs: medical, personal, emotional, and spiritual. *Five Wishes* also encourages discussing your wishes with your family and physician.

Nolo Press
http://nolo.com

Nolo Press publishes "do-it-yourself" legal guides for consumers and small businesses. Founded by legal aid lawyer Jake Warner, it is the nation's oldest and most respected provider of accessible legal information and tools to the general public.

Guides to advanced directives and documents can be downloaded from the website. Useful online articles include *Advance Directives, Living Wills, Power of Attorney: What's The Difference?* by Shae Irving, JD.

RESOURCES FOR RESPIRATORY CARE PRACTITIONERS

The Institute for Rehabilitation Research and Development
The Ottawa Hospital, Ottawa, Canada
http://www.irrd.ca/education/

The Institute for Rehabilitation Research and Development (IRRD) fosters research, development, networking, and the clinical and practical application of rehabilitation for paralytic and neuromuscular diseases. Online education services include protocols and procedures for volume recruitment and secretion mobilization therapies, including mechanical insufflation-exsufflation (MI-E), glossopharyngeal breathing GPB, Cough Assist, lung volume recruitment with resuscitation bag, and mechanical ventilation.

Northwest Assisted Breathing Center
University of Washington Medical Center
1959 Northeast Pacific Street, Box 356522
Seattle, WA 98195
Medical Director: Joshua O. Benditt, MD
E-mail: benditt@u.washington.edu
Lead Respiratory Therapist: Louis Boitano, MS, RRT
E-mail:boitano@u.washington.edu
Identifying Sleep Disordered Breathing in Neuromuscular Disordered
    Patients
http://www.sleepreviewmag.com/issues/articles/2007-01_03.asp
Providing mouth piece ventilation with volume ventilators
http://www.uwtv.org/programs/displayevent.aspx?rID=4123&
    fID=853

Dr. John R. Bach
http://www.doctorbach.com

Professor of Physical Medicine and Rehabilitation, Medical Director of the Center for Ventilator Management Alternatives at University Hospital, Newark, NJ.

Rehabilitation of patients with neuromuscular disease, pulmonary disease, and home mechanical ventilation are the primary clinical focus of Dr. Bach. He has authored more than 250 publications, including seven books on neuromuscular, pulmonary rehabilitation, and noninvasive mechanical ventilation.

His website doctorbach.com includes resources for managing neuromuscular patients, articles on noninvasive ventilation, prevention of respiratory complications, and the hazards of oxygen therapy for neuromuscular disease patients. Available for download are intensive care and outpatient protocols for volume expansion and secretion mobilization techniques. Sample letters of medical necessity for respiratory equipment are available.

RESOURCES FOR HOME CARE PROVIDERS

American Association for Homecare
http://www.aahomecare.org

The American Association for Homecare works to strengthen access to care for people who require medical care in their homes. AA Homecare advocates on behalf of the home care community in legislative and regulatory arenas. AA Homecare provides information about compliance issues, industry trends, data, education and training, networking opportunities, and consumer information.

ETHICAL CONSIDERATIONS IN HEALTH CARE

Vermont Ethics Network
http://www.vtethicsnetwork.org

The Vermont Ethics Network promotes better understanding of ethical issues in modern health care. The organization is dedicated to increasing understanding of ethical issues, values, and choices in health and health care. Its goals include providing education for individuals, care givers, volunteers, policy makers, and communities about ethical issues in health and health care; empowering patients, families, and health professionals to join in constructive dialogue and shared decision making about health values and choices; and engaging policy makers and their constituencies in examining ethical issues embedded in the utilization of health care resources and pursuing an ethically just system of health care for all.

Hastings Center
http://www.thehastingscenter.org

The Hastings Center is an independent, nonpartisan, and nonprofit bioethics research institute founded in 1969 to explore fundamental and emerging questions in medicine, health care, and biotechnology. Much of the Center's research addresses bioethics issues in three broad areas: care and decision making at the end of life, public health priorities, and new and emerging technologies. The center draws on a world-wide network of experts, including an elected association of leading researchers influential in bioethics called Hastings Center Fellows. Interdisciplinary teams frame and examine ethical issues and work to inform professional practice, public conversation, and social policy. The Hastings Center publishes *The Hastings Center Report.*

GENERAL RESOURCES ABOUT ALS

Palliative Care in ALS
David Oliver, MD, Gian Domenico Borasio, MD,
    and Declan Walsh, MD
2000, Oxford University Press
http://www.oup-usa.org

Amyotrophic Lateral Sclerosis: A Guide for Patients and Families
Hiroshi Mitsumoto, MD, and Theodore L. Munsat, MD
2001, Demos Medical Publishing
http://www.demosmedpub.com

Amyotrophic Lateral Sclerosis
Robert Miller, MD, Deborah Gelinas, MD,
    and Patricia O'Connor, RN
2004, Demos Medical Publishing
http://www.demosmedpub.com

Tuesdays with Morrie
Mitch Albom
1997, Doubleday
http://www.randomhouse.com/doubleday

Morrie: In His Own Words
Morrie Schwartz
1999, Walker & Co.

Letting Go: Morrie's Reflections on Living While Dying
1996, Walker & Co.
http://www.walkerbooks.com

Index

251